EATING WELL
FOR
OPTIMUM
HEALTH

*The Essential Guide to Food,
Diet and Nutrition*

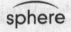

ANDREW WEIL, M.D.

sphere

SPHERE

First published in Great Britain in 2000 by Little, Brown and Company
This edition published in 2001 by Warner Books
Reprinted by Time Warner Paperbacks in 2002
Reprinted by Sphere in 2007
Reissued by Sphere in 2008

11 13 15 14 12 10

Grateful acknowledgment is made to the following for permission to reprint
previously published material:

Ronald E. Koetzsch and Natural Health: Excerpt from "Camaraderie Is the Best Diet" by
Ronald E. Koetzsch (Natural Health, January/February 1994).
Reprinted by permission of the author and Natural Health.

Marlowe & Company, Hodder and Stoughton Limited, and Hodder Headline Australia:
The table, "The Glycemic Index of Some Popular Foods" from The Glucose Revolution by
Jennie Brand-Miller, Ph.D., Thomas M. S. Wolever, M.D., Ph.D., Stephen Colagiuri, M.D.,
and Kaye Foster-Powell, M. Nurt. & Diet. Copyright © 1996, 1998, 1999 by Jennie Brand-
Miller, Ph.D., Thomas M. S. Wolever, M.D., Ph.D., Stephen Colagiuri, M.D., and Kaye
Foster-Powell, M. Nurt. & Diet. Rights in the United Kingdom administered by Hodder and
Stoughton Limited London. Rights in Australia and New Zealand administered by Hodder
Headline Australia, Sydney, from The G.I. Factor: The Glucose Revolution by Jennie Brand-
Miller, Stephen Colagiuri, Kaye Foster-Powell, and Anthony Leeds. Reprinted by permission
of Marlowe & Company, a division of Avalon Publishing Group, Hodder and Stoughton
Limited, and Hodder Headline Australia.

Oldways: The Mediterranean Diet Pyramid developed by Oldways. Copyright © 1994
by Oldways Preservation & Exchange Trust. Reprinted by permission of Oldways,
Cambridge, Mass.

A CIP catalogue record for this book is available from the British Library.

ISBN 978-0-7515-4082-6

Printed and bound in Great Britain by Clays Ltd, St Ives plc

Papers used by Sphere are from well-managed forests
and other responsible sources.

MIX
Paper from
responsible sources
FSC® C104740
www.fsc.org

Sphere
An imprint of
Little, Brown Book Group
100 Victoria Embankment
London EC4Y 0DY

An Hachette UK Company
www.hachette.co.uk

www.littlebrown.co.uk

To my colleagues in Integrative Medicine

CONTENTS

EATING WELL FOR OPTIMUM HEALTH

INTRODUCTION

INTRODUCTION

IN THE COURSE of my work, questions always come up about food and nutrition, diet and health. It is not easy to find the answers to these questions, especially today when we are bombarded by so much confusing and contradictory nutritional information. My purpose in writing this book is to cut through the confusion.

I have always been interested in food, enjoy eating, and have studied the dietary habits of many different cultures around the world, especially to note correlations with patterns of health and illness. As a result of what I have learned, I use dietary change as a primary treatment in my medical practice, and I teach other physicians to do the same.

Throughout my lifetime I have read many words of medical thinking as to what's good for us and what isn't. Not long ago, I read that olive oil was bad for cardiovascular health. Now I see that it is good. I have seen fad diets come and go and then sometimes come again and go again. As I write, low-carbohydrate diets are enjoying a huge wave of popularity. I have serious reservations about them for long-term use . . . but I don't want to get ahead of myself. I will explain the dangers of those diets in due course.

I never want to promise anything I can't deliver, whether in my personal life, in my medical practice, or in my books. I will not make extravagant promises in this book—not of endless life, nor of miracle cures (though diet and nutrition can play a significant role in what I have referred to elsewhere as Spontaneous Healing).

Here is what I *can* promise you in this book:

- I will provide for you all the basic facts of human nutrition.
- I will equip you with the essential information that will allow you to make informed decisions about weight reduction and diet aids.
- I will help you to be able to read labels on all food products, which will allow you to be a far wiser consumer.
- I will discuss a number of popular diets, their pros and cons, and recommend my own diet for optimum health.
- I will provide you with menu plans, recipes, and guidance in eating at home and in restaurants.
- I will give customized dietary advice for a host of common ailments.

It is my sincere belief that if you adhere to the guidelines I have established here you will be the better for it—as will your children—both in the near future and in the years ahead. And just as important as any fact I will demonstrate to you, I want you to emerge from this book clearly convinced that eating for health and eating for pleasure are not incompatible, that it is possible to eat in ways that best serve your body while also getting all the enjoyment you expect from food.

A healthy diet is the cornerstone of a healthy lifestyle. You will find in these pages all the information you need to put that cornerstone in place.

1

THE PRINCIPLES OF
EATING WELL

WHEN I USE the words *eating well,* I mean using food not only to influence health and well-being but to satisfy the senses, providing pleasure and comfort. In addition to supplying the basic needs of the body for calories and nutrients, an optimum diet should also reduce risks of disease and fortify the body's defenses and intrinsic mechanisms of healing. I believe that how we eat is an important determinant of how we feel and how we age. I also believe that food can function as medicine to influence a variety of common ailments.

The American Council on Science and Health, a New York–based nonprofit organization dedicated to "helping distinguish between real and hypothetical health risks," recently suggested ten resolutions for a healthy new year. The council included obvious ones, such as don't smoke, wear seat belts, and install smoke detectors, but addressed diet in only one paragraph:

> *Eat a balanced and varied diet. Avoid obesity and fad diets.* There are no magical guidelines for good nutrition. Patients should resolve to plan their diet around the watchwords "variety, moderation, and balance." Remember: There are no "good" or "bad" foods. The primary danger from food is overindulgence.

I find this advice to be remarkably unhelpful. *Eat a balanced diet?* What is that? I meet people who think that adding a salad with creamy dressing to a cheeseburger and French fries balances the meal. *Avoid obesity?* Sure, that sounds like a good idea, but how do you do it? *There are no "good" or "bad" foods?* What about soybeans? They contain healthy fiber, a fat that may help lower cholesterol, and unusual compounds called isoflavones that may offer significant protection against common forms of cancer. Soybeans seem like a good food to me. What about margarine? For years I've been telling my patients to avoid it because it contains *trans*-fatty acids (TFAs), unnatural fats that promote inflammation, heart disease, and cancer. Sounds like a bad food to me—I won't eat it, even in moderation or in the pursuit of variety.

The primary danger from food is overindulgence? I'm sure my distant ancestors had no problem in that area, but what am I supposed to do when everywhere I look I see tempting offerings of food in ever more novel preparations, when many restaurants score points for the size of portions they serve, when I get more for my money buying giant sizes of food and drink, and when people who love me or want my attention give me food and more food as expressions of their affection or interest?

The poor advice about diet and health that people get far too often when they ask physicians, nurses, registered dietitians, and other representatives of the health-care establishment for help reflects the dearth of good nutritional education in our professional schools. If you look to other sources—alternative practitioners, bookstores, health food stores, the Internet, for example—there is no shortage of information about nutritional influences on health. In fact, there is much too much of it out there, most of it contradictory, unscientific, and intended to promote particular foods, diets, or dietary supplements.

While scanning nutrition-related sites on the Internet, for example, I came across glowing recommendations for products made from "super blue-green algae," microorganisms from a lake in Oregon. I was told that:

> Super Blue Green Algae gives us nutrients and energy at almost no cost to the body's reserves. This algae is 97% assimilable, and many of the nutrients are in forms that are directly usable. For example, the algae's 60% protein content is of a type called glycoproteins, as opposed to the lipoproteins found in vegetables and meat. As a result, the body doesn't have to spend its valuable

resources converting lipoproteins into glycoproteins as it does with other foods. Super Blue Green Algae contains almost every vitamin and mineral needed by the body . . . [and] is one of the richest sources of chlorophyll—a cell regenerator and blood purifier.

Should I rush to order this costly "superfood"? Can it be that all my life my body has been wasting its valuable resources converting lipoproteins to glycoproteins when it could have been getting just what it wanted from pond scum? As for chlorophyll, while it performs a vital function in the life of green plants, it has no role that I know of in human nutrition.

At one extreme are authorities telling us that we are what we eat, that health, good and bad, is entirely or mostly a creation of what we put in our mouths. There is a kernel of attractive logic in that formulation that resonates with common sense. We have to eat to live, because food is fuel for the metabolic engine. The quality of fuel you burn must influence your body, just as the grade of fuel you put into an internal combustion engine influences its performance for better or worse, not only in the short run—a smooth purr versus a ragged knock, for example—but also in the long run, retarding or accelerating the accumulation of deposits that reduce the longevity of valves, rings, and ultimately the entire engine. But it is a long way from this simple observation to the conclusion that diet is everything.

At the other extreme are voices telling us it doesn't matter. "Eat healthy, exercise, die anyway." "Just eat a balanced diet." "My uncle Jake ate big helpings of bacon, eggs, steak, and butter every day of his life and lived to be ninety-nine." "There are no good and bad foods." "People who say you can affect your health and treat disease by changing your diet are food faddists." "It's all in your genes, anyway."

I know of no subject more confused, emotionally charged, and important in our lives than food and nutrition and their influence on our well-being. When I give public talks on health and medicine, the questions I get reveal both the interest and confusion. Here are some examples*:

---

*See Appendix C, page 273, for the answers to these questions.

- How can I lose weight? I've tried everything.
- It seems as if I gain weight just by looking at food. Why?
- I've had cancer. What foods should I avoid?
- I have no energy. Could my diet be the problem?
- I thought we were supposed to avoid dietary fat. Now I'm hearing that fat is okay and carbohydrates are bad. What are the answers?
- Is it okay to eat soybeans if I had breast cancer?
- If I change my diet, can I get off all the drugs I'm taking for my arthritis?
- My five-year-old has asthma. Are there foods he shouldn't be eating? My doctor doesn't seem to know.
- A holistic doctor told me I'm allergic to wheat. What does that mean? I love bread and pasta.
- If I'm eating pretty well, do I need to take vitamins?
- If I'm supposed to be eating more fruits and vegetables, do I have to worry about pesticides on them?
- I don't have time to cook. How can I eat a healthy diet?
- My children like only macaroni and cheese. How can I get them to develop better eating habits?
- I love chocolate. Is it bad for me?
- The cafeteria food at my school is wretched. How can I persuade the school to improve it?
- Is it all right to eat eggs if heart disease runs in your family?
- Is sugar bad for you?
- Are microwave ovens safe?
- Is it dangerous to cook in aluminum pots?
- I read that dairy products could be causing my sinus problems. Isn't milk supposed to be the perfect food?
- Are artificial sweeteners safe?
- Is it okay to drink water with your meals?
- What's the best way to eat if I want to live to be a hundred?

I could extend this list to fill dozens and dozens of pages. It shows the keen interest people have in this subject, their inability to get answers, and their concern about opinions that are contradictory and confusing. People sense the possibility of improving health by making informed choices regarding food, and they sense danger in making uninformed ones, but they do not know where to get information they can trust.

Physicians are at almost the same disadvantage as the rest of us. My medical partner, Dr. Brian Becker, tells me that he was completely turned off the subject of nutrition at the age of ten, when he was forced to listen to a dietitian talk to his fifth-grade class about healthy eating and the four basic food groups then in fashion. "She was overweight, slovenly, smoked at the break, and was in no way anyone I wanted to identify with," he recalls. "Furthermore, the information she gave us was later proved wrong. That one experience stayed with me for years and has made it impossible for me to read or hear anything about nutrition without feeling bored and resentful."

My purpose in writing this book is to explore the issues and controversies surrounding food and nutrition in order to bring clarity to the subject and establish for readers a sense of what eating well means. First I want to state seven basic propositions that underlie my philosophy of food and nutrition and how they both influence health.

WE HAVE TO EAT TO LIVE.

The body requires energy for all of its functions, from the beating of the heart and the elimination of wastes to the transmission of electrical and chemical signals in the nervous system. It gets its energy from food, by taking it in, digesting it, and metabolizing its components. Food is fuel that contains energy from the sun, originally captured and stored by green plants, then passed along to fruits, seeds, and animals. Humans eat these foods, and burn the fuel they contain—that is, combine it with oxygen in a controlled fashion to release and capture the stored solar energy. As long as we live, we have to eat and eat often.

Or do we? Throughout history there have been unsubstantiated reports of persons who survive without eating. Their ability to do so is usually ascribed to sainthood or to mastery of esoteric mental powers.* I can understand that some people are fascinated by the possibility of surviving without eating because of a philosophical quandary: the fact that we live at the expense of other life. Whether we destroy carrots or cows, it is a fact that we are unable to survive and grow without ending the existence of other life-forms; "nature red in tooth and claw" includes us. (Green plants, of course, are not

*See Appendix D, page 278, for more on this subject.

burdened with this requirement: They eat light, binding the energy of photons from the sun into chemical bonds that forge carbon dioxide and water into glucose, the simple sugar that is the most basic foodstuff. They can later burn this glucose as fuel or convert it into starch or fat for storage.)

In my case and for most of us the reality is that we must eat to live, usually several times a day. Not having enough food is seen as an ultimate misfortune and a cause of human suffering, and having it in abundance is cause for rejoicing.

EATING IS A MAJOR SOURCE OF PLEASURE.

In societies where food is scarce, it is seen primarily as a necessity of life and little thought is given to it beyond that. In societies where food is abundant, people use it for purposes far beyond mere survival. In our society, a great deal of time, energy, and money goes into the preparation and consumption of food that is intended to provide pleasure. Gastronomic pleasure is complex, however. We respond not only to the odors, tastes, and textures of food but to its associations. Think of the comfort foods you would turn to if you were sick, hurt, or sad. Would you choose a baked potato? buttered toast? a steak? ice cream? Do you associate comfort with foods that a caring parent brought you when you were sick in childhood: chicken soup or rice pudding, for example? The appearance and smell of such food combines with its taste and feel in the mouth to create a pleasurable experience that also includes satisfaction at being nourished.

I respond positively to food prepared with care and attention and negatively to food that is careless and artless. When I am traveling and go into a strange restaurant, I can often tell at once whether food will be good by the feel of the place. I have found wonderful food in simple, inexpensive establishments and disappointing food in many expensive ones. The simplest meals can be extraordinarily satisfying if they are prepared and served with care and with the intention to provide pleasure as well as sustenance. And I have observed that when truly wonderful food is served to a group of diners, conversation virtually stops, and people concentrate almost entirely on the pleasure of eating.

Psychologists describe food as a primary reinforcer—that is, something with intrinsic power to shape behavior. Give an animal food when it exhibits a certain behavior, and it will behave that way more frequently. Food is an especially powerful reinforcer, used by trainers to elicit performances of animals in circuses and movies in apparent contrast to their wild natures. In order for food to exert this effect, it must be presented to an animal that is hungry. In other words, a state of relative deprivation of the reinforcing stimulus must exist for it to exert its power over behavior. If an animal is sated it is in a refractory state, not responsive to the reinforcing stimulus of food.

Everyone knows the equivalent human state, when deprivation makes food so appealing that we would do almost anything to get it. A quirk of the human condition is that the imagined pleasure of consuming food that is not there often exceeds the actual pleasure of consuming food that is.

Pleasure we experience in our minds must also be in our brains. Neuroscientists have identified a number of systems in the brain that correlate with pleasurable experience, focusing especially on the neurotransmitters dopamine, serotonin, and noradrenalin. Disturbances in these systems may be associated with addiction, risk-seeking behavior, and the calamitous symptom of *anhedonia,* the inability to experience pleasure that often accompanies severe depression. The identification of imbalances in neurotransmitters and their receptors on neurons opened the way to inventions of new psychopharmaceutical drugs that are now widely prescribed to correct the imbalances with variable clinical success.

It may well be that all addictive behavior has common correlates in neuroreceptor physiology and that we will one day understand this physiology well enough to treat addiction effectively by means of drugs. What is certain, however, is that addictive behavior can form around all pleasurable experiences, eating among them. People who develop addictive patterns of eating are often trying to reduce anxiety, alleviate depression, anesthetize themselves, or otherwise manipulate their psychophysical states, because food and eating modify neurochemistry, including that of brain centers regulating pleasure, arousal, and mood. Looking at addictive eating in this way makes it appear more understandable yet more complex than simple craving or failure of willpower.

Most of us know people who eat immoderately, although many food addicts may conceal their behavior and indulge themselves in private. Here is a snapshot of one prodigious eater, the writer A. J. Liebling, provided by his fellow writer and friend Brendan Gill in his memoir *Here at The New Yorker*:

> It is said to be a weakness in my character not to be much interested in food, and Liebling was a true trencherman, whose appetite astonished and appalled me. I saw that he was, in the old saying, digging his grave with his teeth, but there was nothing to be done about it; the pleasure he took in gourmandizing was obviously identical to the pleasure other people took in listening to a Chopin nocturne. One day at lunch at the Villa Nova, during a period when, on doctor's orders, Liebling was making a valiant effort to eat lightly, he ordered a succulent dish of veal, peppers, and eggplant, which, in the Villa Nova tradition, arrived at the table aswim and asizzle in a large pewter platter. Liebling quickly polished off the entire platter, then, breaking chunks of bread from a long loaf on the table, soaked up the remaining gravy, all but literally licking the platter clean. It was a meal the very thought of which was enough to keep me from feeling hungry for a week. Liebling beckoned to the waiter. I thought he would be asking for the check, but not at all. "I'll have one more of the same," he said.

Obviously, not all of us respond to food in the same way. Although it acts as a primary reinforcer for everyone who is hungry, individuals derive various degrees of pleasure from it. For some, eating is mostly a necessity of life; attention paid to the sensual aspect of food is minimal, and pleasure is sought elsewhere—in listening to music or in sex, for example. Nonetheless, I think it is fair to say that food is an important source of pleasure for most of us, and a primary source of it for some of us. For that reason, any recommendations for healthy eating that diminish or eliminate the pleasure of the experience of eating are certain to fail.

FOOD THAT IS HEALTHY AND FOOD THAT GIVES PLEASURE ARE NOT MUTUALLY EXCLUSIVE.

A common lament I hear from patients is, "Everything I like to eat is bad for me." This is often paired with a question: "If it's bad for you, why does it taste so good?" Actually, as I will soon explain, there are perfectly good reasons why our senses guide us to foods high in fat and sugar, to large portions of meat, to fast food, and to what even those who love it characterize as "junk food." The fault is not with our taste but in the way we have changed the environment to make once scarce foods readily available.

A more puzzling question is, "Why is healthy food so dull?" I have my own answer to that one, which is that many people who preach the virtues of healthy eating do not really like food, or, more precisely, are not the people who are neurochemically programmed to derive significant pleasure from the experience of eating. Many writers of diet books are in this category as are many nutritionists, dietitians, and health professionals who tell others how they should eat. They are not lovers of good food.

Consider this recipe for Sun Garden Burgers from a book of "simple recipes for living well":

> Combine carrot pulp [leftover residue after juicing carrots], ground flax and sunflower seeds, finely minced celery, onion, parsley, and red pepper; season with soy sauce; shape into patties and leave them in the sun until warm or place in warm oven for 15 minutes. These are delicious served in a cabbage leaf "bun": fold a cabbage leaf over the burger with any condiments you like or cut two squares of cabbage from the large leaves and place the burger in between them.

I rest my case.

Years ago, when I was first experimenting with vegetarian cooking, I had an English couple as houseguests. I served them a meal of whole grains and, I thought, artfully prepared vegetables. They ate it with curiosity and mild enthusiasm, but when one of them came to breakfast the next morning, he said with a wry face and one hand on his stomach, "Health food really gives you gas, doesn't it?"

If your main experience of healthy food is that it gives you gas, you are not likely to come back for more. Or, if you do, you must be one of those who find virtue in suffering, convinced that health and pleasure do not come together at the table.

My job is to convince you otherwise. I like food. I experience pleasure from eating, and I am unwilling to sacrifice that experience in a quest for better health. I have spent years studying the medical literature on nutrition, working with patients who need to improve their diets, exploring the cuisines of other cultures, and testing and devising recipes that conform to healthy guidelines. My conviction is that healthy food and delicious food are not mutually exclusive; the concept of "eating well" must embrace both the health-promoting and pleasure-giving aspects of food. This is the most important assumption underlying the philosophy of this book. If you have had dreadful encounters with health food, if it has given you gas or worse, I can assure you that I will show you how to change your diet in ways that will move you toward optimum health and longevity without your having to give up everything you like to eat.

EATING IS AN IMPORTANT FOCUS OF SOCIAL INTERACTION.

Coming together to share food is a behavioral pattern we have in common with many other creatures. The word *companion* derives from the Latin word for bread, *panis*. Breaking bread together both establishes and symbolizes a fundamental social bond. A Japanese phrase for an intimate companion is "one who eats rice from the same bowl."

Think of the elaborate rituals of communal eating that have evolved from the simple act of sharing the most basic foodstuffs. Think of the service industries that have developed to provide us with power breakfasts, business lunches, and romantic dinners. Consider the communal feasts that punctuate the calendars of the world's religions. In fact, the words *festive, festival,* and *feast* have a common Latin root, suggesting that occasions merry, joyous, and significant are all distinguished by eating in company.

The social importance of food and eating, like their association with pleasure, must be honored by anyone advocating eating well. Too often people who follow rigid diets in the name of health isolate themselves from the social interaction that is itself an important factor in optimum health. I can think of no better illustration of this observation than this excerpt from an article entitled, "Camaraderie Is the Best Diet," by Ronald Koetzsch that appeared in *Natural Health* magazine:

I spent a month in Russia, teaching at Moscow State University. One weekend, Martha (my teaching partner) and I went with several Russian students to visit St. Petersburg. . . . We arrived around

11:00 p.m. Our hosts were a baby-faced medical student and his wife, and they had prepared a Russian banquet for us. There was borscht, thick slabs of dark bread, mounds of butter, salted fish, apples, pastry, cheese, and vodka. By the time we sat down to eat, it was well past midnight. . . .

I was tired and not particularly hungry. And I remembered that eating late usually makes me feel lethargic and dull in the morning. Like Buddhist monks who do not eat after midday, I prefer to go to bed on an empty stomach.

So when the eating began, I politely explained that I wasn't feeling well and that I would just have some water and apple juice. My hostess said, "If you don't feel well, the answer is to eat. Yes. Yes. Eat for health." . . .

I held to abstinence, though, with a slight sense of self-righteousness. While everyone else, including Martha, ate, drank, and was merry, I sipped juice and water and waited for the moment when I could politely excuse myself and go to bed. After an hour or so, I did, but the eating, drinking, conversation, and laughter continued long thereafter. One of my last thoughts before sleep was: "Well I, anyway, will be clear and energetic tomorrow when we tour the city."

Alas, such was not the case. I was groggy and out of sorts, and I felt alienated from the others. And they, despite going to bed full of food and vodka, were cheerful and brimming with energy.

I was a bit dismayed by the apparent injustice. . . .

Soon after my Russian sojourn, I was in Germany . . . visiting a friend in a village near Kassel, and we attended a breakfast marking the end of a local holiday. The meal was served in a huge hall. In the middle was a 30-piece German brass band playing "oom-pah-pah" music at a mind-numbing volume. Hundreds of men dressed in dark suits and frilled white shirts were sitting at long tables, drinking beer, talking, laughing, and occasionally breaking into song.

As soon as I sat down, a large mug of frothy beer was placed before me, and my immediate neighbors—red-faced and smiling—raised their mugs in salute . . . it did not seem a time to ask for peppermint tea. . . . [I] took a sip of my beer. It was thick and delicious. I took another sip and started talking to my neighbor, a policeman from the town. When I finished my mug, another appeared in front of me. . . .

Eventually, breakfast was served. It featured a deep-fried pork cutlet about the size of a Frisbee. To one who has eaten little meat and no pork for over two decades, it seemed "The Mother of All Pork Cutlets" . . . what was I to do?—ask our Walkyrie of a waitress to bring my hummus and alfalfa sprout sandwich instead? I dug in, eating the cutlet, potato salad, and everything else on the plate with relish. It was delicious.

When we left, I was relaxed, happy, and so alert that I noticed the floor and other parts of the seemingly solid German building were actually moving. I had a sense of foreboding, though. When will the ax of judgment fall upon my dietary sins? I wondered. But it never did. I felt unusually energetic and ebullient that whole day and for days afterward. . . . I look forward to my next breakfast of beer, pork cutlet, and song.

Koetzsch's conclusion is that when "food is blessed by being shared, by being eaten in fellowship amidst conversation and laughter . . . all food is 'health' food." I agree.

HOW WE EAT REFLECTS AND DEFINES OUR PERSONAL AND CULTURAL IDENTITY.

On Thursday nights, people throughout Sweden sit down to the same meal, beginning with a thick soup made from yellow split peas. They take pleasure and comfort both in the food and in the knowledge that they are joining their countrymen and women in a national ritual that transcends both space and time—their grandparents and great-grandparents ate this weekly meal as well. Eating particular foods thus helps define identity and membership in ethnic and national groups and in family.

Ritual meals featuring special foods help renew bonds between friends, family members, and communities on both sacred and secular feast days. Consider the Jewish Passover seder, where those in attendance ask and answer questions about the special items on the menu. "Why on this night do we eat only unleavened bread [*matzoh*], when on all other nights we eat either leavened or unleavened bread?" The answer reminds the diners of their distant ancestors who labored as slaves in Egypt and had to flee so quickly that they could not allow the dough for their bread to rise. A delicious spread, *charoset*, made of finely chopped walnuts and apples, moistened with sweet wine, and often flavored with cinnamon, appears only at the seder. It symbolizes the mortar used by the enslaved Israelites to construct the Pharaoh's buildings. Participants eat some of it spread on matzoh with a topping of pungent horseradish—sometimes so pungent that it brings tears to the eyes. This combination, said to be the invention of Rabbi Hillel, a great Jewish sage who lived around the time of Jesus, is supposed to remind those who eat it of the inseparability of sweetness and bitterness, of joy and sorrow, in human life. Passover and Easter both evolved from older pagan festivals celebrating the return of light and life at the spring equinox. Hard-boiled eggs appear on tables at both holidays because eggs are symbols of fertility and renewal, as do spring greens as symbols of new growth.

Special foods are also prominent at secular celebrations of the new year in cultures around the world. If you are Japanese, this most important holiday of the year, when you would clean your house from top to bottom and visit, and be visited by, friends and relatives, would feature the preparation and eating of *mochi*, a sticky treat made from glutinous sweet rice, traditionally and laboriously prepared in company by soaking, steaming, and pounding it in huge mortars with wooden clubs. (Electric countertop *mochi* makers, a recent invention, have made the process effortless and taken away some of the power of the ritual.) In the American South, the special dish is often boiled black-eyed peas, supposed to bring good luck for the coming year.

Of course, identity defined and secured by food and eating habits has as much to do with forbidden and disliked foods as with those that are enjoyed and promoted. Orthodox Jews will not eat pork. Orthodox Hindus will not eat meat. Orthodox Muslims do not consume alcohol. Food taboos are common, sometimes elaborate, and oftentimes genuine attempts to connect to, and respect, religious beliefs and traditions. On the other hand, some food taboos seem ridiculous. And the taboos of one group may strike another group as most peculiar, emphasizing the "otherness" of those who refuse to eat fish, fowl, garlic, or sugar, for example. And so identity is further strengthened by defining oneself and one's culture or social group as different through eating or not eating what other people eat.

Most readers of this book will shun insects as food, regarding peoples who eat them as very different, indeed. The relish with which Australian aborigines eat witchetty grubs, the fat larvae of cossid moths, is a sure sign of their differentness and primitiveness. But if we want to be accepted by other people on their territory, we may have to swallow our aversions. My friend Wade Davis, a fellow alumnus of ethnobotanical training at the Harvard Botanical Museum, has made a career of studying and writing about native peoples throughout the world. His success stems, in part, from a noteworthy ability to win the trust of others. He says, "It can be as simple as willingness to eat what's put in front of you. If you walk into an Indian village and say, 'I'm sorry, I don't eat grubs,' well, that's going to create a barrier."

Conversely, barriers may be reinforced when people from one culture move to foreign territory and consume foods their new neighbors shun. In the Western world dogs are not considered food, because people identify with them, value them as pets, and appreciate their qualities of intelligence, affection, and loyalty. But in some parts of Asia people like to eat dogs, some of which—young, black dogs, for example—are considered especially delicious and nourishing. When large numbers of immigrants from Southeast Asia came to the United States in the wake of the Vietnam War, this dietary difference created bitter friction. Residents of California did not react well to the new arrivals' penchant for nabbing and eating their pets, surely a sign of a "barbaric" culture.*

The power of food to define social and cultural identity may also depend on particular ingredients, combinations of ingredients, or preparations that provide instantly recognizable textures, flavors, and aromas. The steamed rice of Japan that sticks together and has a subtle, earthy flavor is nothing like the steamed rice of India, whose grains are separate, drier, and more aromatic. *Poi,* the sour, pasty staple made from taro root, is a unique food of Hawaii and related cultures of Oceania. Lemongrass, chile, mint, and garlic occur together only in the cuisines of Southeast Asia. Olive oil, tomatoes, garlic, and basil create a signature flavor of the cooking of southern Italy, while olive oil, lemon juice, garlic, mint, and cumin in combination announce the Middle Eastern origin of a dish, and tomato, peanuts, and chile are a characteristic flavor principle of West African cuisine.

---

*Of course, the ultimate food taboo is against eating one's own kind. Many animals observe it, as do most humans. Authorities differ about the existence of human societies that practice cannibalism regularly rather than as isolated incidents, but it is clear that many societies have attributed the practice to others.

Often, it is these culture-specific tastes, odors, and textures that people long for when they have left their native lands and that occasion
such joy when people reconnect with them. The French pine for their
excellent bread when they travel in other countries, Indians for their
curries, Japanese for their rice. And often, when people have aban-
doned their traditional foods, whether by choice or by circumstance,
they will seek them out again when they are sick, infirm, or otherwise
in need. For example, I am told that it is common for Japanese who
have long eaten Western diets to come back to meals of fish, rice, vegetables, and miso soup in their old age. Perhaps their digestive systems are better adapted to these dishes or perhaps the associations of
the foods, their reinforcing of cultural identity, is comforting.

I present these ideas to point out another obstacle to motivating
people to change their eating habits in order to improve health. There
is a great deal of psychological, social, and cultural investment in
what we eat, and unless this aspect of food is acknowledged, change
will not be possible. Let me give a few examples of the problem. In
India, a principal cooking fat is *ghee,* a form of clarified butter—that
is, butter that has been heated and strained to remove milk solids.
Ghee has a distinctive, nutty flavor appealing to both Indians and
Westerners and is more stable than butter; it can be stored unrefriger-
ated. It is also pure butterfat, the most saturated of dietary fats, and a
major contributor to atherosclerosis and coronary heart disease,
rates of which are currently very high in India. But it won't do simply
to tell Indians that ghee is unhealthy and that they should switch to
olive oil. As a product of the cow, ghee is regarded as a blessing from
the gods by Hindus, who use it in religious rites, among other things,
to anoint sacred objects. How could such a holy substance be harmful to the body? Hindus ask. Besides, olive oil tastes funny to them,
especially in curry.

Many Japanese do not care for the flavor of olive oil either, but
their traditional diet is so low in both total fat and saturated fat that
they need not worry on that score. Where they could do better is in
consumption of the fiber in whole grains, since their staple, white
rice, provides very little. Most Japanese resist eating brown rice,
however, for several reasons. They have long regarded it as a food of
the lower social classes, much as Europeans used to look down on
whole-grain bread as peasant food. In addition, during World War II,
when white rice was hard to get, many families ate brown rice as a

scarcity food, so it has a further negative association for the older generation. Finally, many Japanese believe their intestinal tracts are shorter and more delicate than those of Westerners and hence less able to process "rough" foods like unpolished grains. It does not help that brown rice is a favorite food of hippies, followers of macrobiotics, and other—to them—dietary extremists.

Nor is it easy to persuade Americans to eat tofu or bean curd, a classic and beloved food of Japan, China, and Korea. Made from soy milk by a process analogous to making fresh farmer's cheese from cow's milk, tofu is a good protein source, with a far healthier fat than butterfat and a good measure of soy isoflavones, compounds that appear to offer significant protection to women against breast cancer and to men against prostate cancer. Some of the American resistance to tofu is simple neophobia, fear of novel foods, but besides that, in its more common forms, tofu has a very bland taste and a squishy texture that Americans find unappealing. Japanese love the delicate flavor and custardlike texture of freshly made tofu. They flock to famous, centuries-old tofu restaurants in Kyoto to eat blocks of it, steamed over hot water, with no flavoring other than a bit of soy sauce and fresh ginger. I have known many American housewives who have read of the health benefits of tofu, bought cartons of it in grocery stores, and attempted to serve it as is to their families with disastrous results. Kids put it directly into the "yuck" pile, and husbands wouldn't touch it.

There are ways around these obstacles if you recognize them. The suggestion can be made to Indians that ghee is terrific for rubbing on things, including the skin, but that it should be ingested in moderation, perhaps added in small quantities to healthier oils as a flavoring. Japanese can be encouraged to try forms of rice that are *somewhat* polished—light brown rice—or to eat mixtures of white and brown rice or to introduce brown rice into the diet gradually. As for tofu, it can be made into dishes that Americans like by disguising it with familiar flavors and textures. I've tasted a delicious nondairy chocolate cream pie made from tofu, for example, as well as a robust Italian-style pasta sauce made with ground, sautéed tofu instead of ground meat. Most Americans who were served these dishes would never suspect they were eating bean curd.

Eating well means, among other things, not rejecting or giving up the characteristics of cuisine that help define oneself or one's society but rather adapting them to conform to dietary principles that promote optimum health.

HOW WE EAT IS ONE DETERMINANT OF HEALTH.

I have already indicated my belief that, just as the quality of fuel influences the performance and longevity of an internal combustion engine, so the quality of food we eat must influence the life and health of the body. The question is how great that influence is relative to other factors. In the heading above I want to emphasize the word *one*. The determinants of health are myriad, starting with genetics and including a great many environmental, psychosocial, and spiritual factors. Diet is only one aspect of lifestyle, and lifestyle is only one set of variables in the mix. It is probably not possible to isolate from this complexity any one element and specify its exact contribution to health. Certainly, it is false to claim, as some do, that diet is the sole or most important determinant of health, or, as the cliché says, that we are what we eat.

Nevertheless, it is possible to get an idea of the influence of diet by looking at the effects of dietary change in large populations and through epidemiology, the study of the incidence and frequency of diseases in populations.

For example, during World War II, deaths from heart attacks dropped precipitously in Denmark, Holland, and other occupied countries of Western Europe, when popular foods high in saturated fat—butter, cheese, and meat, especially—became scarce or unobtainable. When those foods reappeared on tables after the war, deaths from heart attacks rose to previous rates. Japanese women on traditional diets have one of the lowest rates of breast cancer in the world, but when they move to America and eat like Americans, their breast cancer risk quickly rises. Japanese men on traditional diets have low rates of prostate cancer compared to American men, and when they do get it, their tumors behave much less aggressively than those of Americans. At present, Japan and China are both in the midst of sweeping dietary change, in which traditional patterns of eating are weakening in the face of shifts to Western diets, with greatly increased consumption of beef, dairy products, and even American-type fast food. Already rates of "Western diseases" like atherosclerosis and coronary heart disease, once rare in East Asia, are rising.

These countries are living laboratories in which we are able to observe correlations between changes in diet and changes in health. Similarly, subgroups with different eating habits may have very different health problems from the larger societies in which they live. Studies of Seventh Day Adventists in America, a vegetarian Christian sect, show them to have much lower rates of cardiovascular disease than other Americans. Still, the exact contribution of vegetarianism to this difference is not clear, because Seventh Day Adventists also do not smoke or drink alcohol, and they enjoy the psychosocial support of a cohesive community that many other Americans lack.

At the University of Arizona's Program in Integrative Medicine, I teach doctors and other health professionals lifestyle medicine, which has a strong preventive orientation and encourages patients to change their habits before disease appears. Our physicians are taught to take dietary histories of all patients as well as to inquire about such things as their uses of dietary supplements and mood-altering drugs (including alcohol and caffeine); patterns of exercise; relationships with spouses, children, parents, friends, and coworkers; sources of stress in their lives and ways they deal with it; sources of strength, including religion and spirituality; patterns of rest and sleep. My colleagues and I evaluate this information in the context of the patients' past medical histories, family histories, and present symptoms, if any. I have found this approach to be invaluable in dealing with common health risks and problems, and I regret that in conventional medical settings today, few physicians have time to ask these questions or analyze the answers. Profit-driven health maintenance organizations (HMOs) do not want to "waste" doctors' valuable time in this way.

Diet has special significance among lifestyle factors in that people have total control over it, at least potentially. You cannot change your genes, control the quality of the air you breathe all the time, or avoid the stresses of everyday life, but you can decide what to eat and what not to eat, even if you are stuck on occasion in an institutional cafeteria. It is a shame not to take advantage of that control by making wise choices from what is available and by informing yourself about wise and unwise choices of food.

My conclusion is that diet is an important influence on health, one that you can control to a greater degree than other factors, and that eating a good diet does not excuse you from attending to other aspects of lifestyle if you want to enjoy optimum health.

CHANGING HOW WE EAT IS ONE STRATEGY FOR MANAGING DISEASE AND RESTORING HEALTH.

In the fifth century B.C., Hippocrates, the godfather of Western medicine, advised people to "let food be your medicine and medicine be your food." This idea is not much in fashion in the West today, but it is strikingly current in Asia. In both India and China, for example, highly developed systems of healing and cuisine are intertwined. Dietary modification is a primary therapeutic intervention in Ayurvedic medicine as well as in traditional Chinese medicine, and in both Indian and Chinese cooking, ingredients are valued for their health-promoting properties as much as for their flavors.

Ginger, popular in both cultures, is esteemed by Chinese cooks for its ability to neutralize noxious qualities of flesh foods and to stimulate the stomach, and by Indian cooks for its warming and gas-dispelling effects. Its medicinal virtues—ginger is a powerful anti-inflammatory agent as well as an excellent remedy for stomach upset—are just being rediscovered by Westerners. Turmeric, responsible for the yellow color of curries, is another effective anti-inflammatory herb, prized by Indians for its healing properties at least as much as for its taste and color. An extract of it called curcumin is now available in capsules in health food stores here, and people are taking it for the treatment of arthritis and other inflammatory disorders.

This blurring of lines between foods and medicines that is common throughout Asia has produced an interesting tradition of healing cuisine in that part of the world: specific recipes for specific complaints that can be prepared at home but are also offered at specialty restaurants. Nina Simonds, an expert on Asian cooking, has described a visit to one of these establishments in her book *A Spoonful of Ginger*:

> I was seated in front of Mr. Li Xian Xing, a Chinese herbalist who was trying to diagnose my malady. I complained that I had no appetite and that I was constantly cold. He checked the pulse of my right hand; it was weak and slow. He inspected my tongue and noticed that it was pale and slightly white. He made his diagnosis. "You are too yin," he solemnly pronounced, and prescribed an order of baked lamb with Chinese wolfberries and a pot of "double-boiled" chicken soup (two yang dishes).

This was no ordinary herbalist's office, although I was surrounded by Chinese herbs. We were seated at the front of the Imperial Herbal restaurant in Singapore, where Mr. Li is the resident herbalist. From the day it first opened . . . the Imperial Herbal has drawn praise from its local and international clientele for its masterful marriage of herbs and Chinese haute cuisine. And Mr. Li has acquired a devoted following of customers who come to the restaurant for treatment. I had come to be treated for a minor ailment and to sample the legendary food. . . .

The chefs not only create their own specialties but also adapt classic dishes to make them even healthier: Beggar's Chicken—an eastern specialty where a whole chicken is first stuffed and wrapped in a lotus leaf, then surrounded by clay and baked for several hours before the clay is cracked open at the table—is embellished further with the addition of four yin herbs and four yang herbs to reinforce blood and energy. Lacquered Peking Duck is served with paper-thin homemade Mandarin pancakes enriched with a flavorless herb that reduces cholesterol.

The list of soups is especially impressive: Double-boiled Soft-Shell River Turtle Soup is a yin energy tonic that, according to the menu, strengthens the body's immune system and helps to prevent cancer. Chicken Soup with Wolfberry promotes blood circulation, and Freshwater Fish with American Ginseng promotes the energy to offset fatigue and "shortness of breath."

Here is Hippocrates's advice put into full practice. Americans have no therapeutic restaurants to go to, and their doctors, while they might approve of Mom's chicken soup for a cold, rarely think about using food as medicine and medicine as food. Things are different at our Integrative Medicine clinic. We do not yet have our own restaurant, but our doctors routinely ask patients to change their diets—to eliminate some foods and add others—as one strategy for managing their conditions. Just as diet is only one factor influencing health, so dietary change is only one therapeutic approach, never recommended in isolation. Our patients also get prescriptions for exercise, relaxation training, dietary supplements, and botanical remedies, as well as referrals to both conventional and alternative practitioners for further diagnostic evaluations and treatments. When they get better, we cannot specify the exact contribution of dietary change to the favorable outcome, but often we regard it as significant.

Recently, I saw a seventy-year-old woman with lifelong asthma who had access to the best conventional medical care in the country and was dependent on a great deal of suppressive and toxic medication. She had an exemplary lifestyle and wanted to know if integrative medicine had anything to offer her. Her dietary history revealed high consumption of dairy products, and when I asked about this, she told me she had grown up on a farm in Wisconsin, had always loved milk, cheese, and yogurt, and had never been told that milk could aggravate asthma. I also discovered that she had a strongly allergic history, including infantile eczema, often a sign of milk intolerance. At the top of my list of recommendations to her, I wrote, "Eliminate all milk and milk products from your diet. You can substitute soy or rice milk, nondairy frozen desserts, cheese substitutes made from soy or almonds." The patient knew this was going to be a challenge: "Those are my main foods," she said.

Nevertheless, she made the adjustment, and although I told her not to expect to see the full effect of the change for two months, she noted improvement after only a few weeks and subsequently had one of her best winters ever, winter usually being her worst time of year. She found it incredible that no doctor, in all the years she had sought medical attention, had made this dietary suggestion to her.

Many patients who come to our clinic have inflammatory diseases: arthritis, tendinitis, lupus, and other autoimmune disorders. As part of a comprehensive treatment program, we recommend changes in dietary fats to manipulate the body's control of inflammation. (In its place, inflammation is a mechanism of the body's healing system that increases circulation and immune activity at sites of injury and infection. Out of place or when persistent, inflammation is a problem, a symptom of imbalance of the hormones that control it.) The major hormones that can increase or decrease inflammation are called prostaglandins; the body synthesizes them from fatty acids. Depending on which fatty acids predominate in the diet, this synthesis can favor pro- or anti-inflammatory prostaglandins, creating a therapeutic opportunity through dietary change. If you eat a lot of safflower oil, sunflower oil, corn oil, or sesame oil, or products made from them, or margarine, vegetable shortening, or products made from them or from other partially hydrogenated oils, the synthetic pathway will produce more of the prostaglandins that increase inflammation. If you avoid those fats and instead eat olive oil, walnuts, flax or hemp oil, and such oily fish as salmon, sardines, herring, and mackerel, your body will instead produce more of the anti-inflammatory hormones, with obvious beneficial results on inflamed tissues.

This therapeutic approach is an example of nutritional medicine, a subject not currently taught in medical schools, one central to the Integrative Medicine that I promote, and one sure to come into its own in coming years, because it opens so many therapeutic possibilities with little or none of the toxicity associated with pharmaceutical drugs. Later, I will outline how the principles of nutritional medicine can be applied, giving recommendations for the management of common ailments using food as medicine.* It is my hope that doctors of the future will begin to honor the wisdom of the past and once again use food as medicine.

Here, to review, are the seven basic principles of diet and health that provide a foundation for building a system of practical nutrition and coming to an understanding of the meaning of eating well:

- We have to eat to live.
- Eating is a major source of pleasure.
- Food that is healthy and food that gives pleasure are not mutually exclusive.
- Eating is an important focus of social interaction.
- How we eat reflects and defines our personal and cultural identity.
- How we eat is one determinant of health.
- Changing how we eat is one strategy for managing disease and restoring health.

I will now review some of the big questions about diet and health, summarizing what we know scientifically about the components of our diets and how they impact our health, for better or for worse.

*See Appendix B, page 264.

A HEALING STORY:
FROM FRENCH FRIES TO KALE

KEN ROSEN at thirty-one is just finishing his studies in New York to become a practitioner of traditional Chinese medicine, a major change of direction from an early career as a filmmaker. His interest in health and healthful eating developed slowly and steadily over a number of years. Here is his story:

I was raised on a diet of French fries and grilled cheese sandwiches. Somewhere along the way, my mom introduced whole wheat bread and a few other health food items. I didn't like them.

At age twelve, I was diagnosed with Hodgkin's disease. I underwent a number of lymph node biopsies, had my spleen removed, and was treated with radiation. The doctors told me I was cured but would have to take penicillin for the rest of my life in order to make up for the loss of my spleen as part of my immune system. I took penicillin until I was sixteen, then, on instinct and over the objections of my doctors, I discontinued it. I made an effort to eat better. Then someone told me about echinacea, and I began using it whenever I felt a cold coming on. It worked great—kept me from getting really sick—and opened my mind to the effectiveness of natural medicine.

When I was studying film production at New York University, I mostly ate take-out and restaurant food, whatever I could get. I was in the film business for four years, directing and writing. Then in 1994 I got thyroid cancer—a direct result of the radiation treatment for Hodgkin's. I had to have a total thyroidectomy. That was a real wake-up call to take charge of my life, especially my diet.

After I recovered I went to India and for the first time focused on the fact that other cultures exist, that there is more than one perspective. When I came back, I knew I wanted to be a health professional. I considered medical school and naturopathic medical school, then settled on studying Chinese medicine because of the appeal of its philosophy, especially its emphasis on balance and change. I started at a school in San Diego and later transferred to one in Manhattan.

I tried to learn as much as I could about diet and health but was discouraged by all the crazy ideas out there. I started cutting down on animal products, eating more leafy greens and whole grains. I went through a period of intellectualizing my food, classifying everything as good or bad. I think that was a mistake. I think you should just enjoy food but also ask yourself whether you really have an appetite for it. And you have to allow time to digest it.

I taught myself to cook. I found it easy to cook for other people, but it took me two years to learn to cook for myself and enjoy it. It's been a real lesson for me, finding out that I can nourish myself.

Americans need to eat a more cleansing diet. We're especially top-heavy in processed foods as opposed to whole foods and in doughy, bready things. And we eat huge portions of everything, especially meat. My experience in India gave me this perspective on our eating habits here. There are days to feast and days to eat really simple food. Some days I'll just eat big bowls of steamed kale.

I feel strong and healthy, and I look forward to using nutritional medicine in my practice after I graduate this spring. My favorite new meal—you'll love this—is a huge pile of steamed kale with little strips of broiled filet mignon on top—amazing!

A HEALING STORY:
THE KNIFE AND FORK
ARE POWERFUL TOOLS

MEL ZUCKERMAN is the founder of Canyon Ranch, a premier health spa, with branches in Lenox, Massachusetts, and Las Vegas in addition to the original Tucson, Arizona, facility. A successful real-estate developer and heavy meat eater, his conversion to a good diet and healthy lifestyle happened suddenly. Here's his story:

I was always thirty to forty pounds overweight from my thirties on. I also had hypertension that ran on my father's side of the family, got an ulcer in my twenties, and had lifelong asthma that interfered with physical activity. The doctors I saw just told me to lose weight but never told me how to keep it off, and they never gave me a sense that I could exercise. My encounters with the medical profession in those days were not very empowering.

I tried all sorts of diets, but then I'd go back to the way I always ate, a real yo-yo pattern. When I turned forty, I had a general health and fitness assessment. The doctor told me there was nothing specifically wrong but that my body was that of someone twenty-five to thirty years older. That stayed in my mind, but I didn't do anything about it until ten years later when my father died from lung cancer six months after he was diagnosed. He was a smoker, and watching him in those last six months, hearing him say he wished he had lived differently, gave me the motivation to change. So when I turned fifty, I spent four weeks at a spa in California.

That was in 1978. Twenty months later I opened Canyon Ranch in Tucson.

My main reason for opening a spa was that I wanted to continue to live the healthy lifestyle I had learned in California and make it available to my friends. Originally, Canyon Ranch was an innovative fat farm with an emphasis on the whole person. We relied on registered dietitians and exercise physiologists from the very start, always making nutrition a centerpiece of our programs.

When I began cutting way down on meat and fat, eating more fruits and vegetables, and exercising regularly, I started to have much more energy. I was able to keep my weight under control for the first time. The exercise was a great boost for my self-esteem. I was able to reach levels of physicality I never dreamed would be possible even when I was in my teens. I took up jogging and even ran a couple of marathons in my fifties.

But as I got into my later sixties, I noticed a change. I had more difficulty maintaining my desired weight and experienced more mood swings. I was prone to depression for much of my life, and it started getting worse. What I've done that has made a big difference is to cut down on carbohydrates. I'd been eating a lot of bread and pasta. Now I eat pasta rarely, consume much less bread, and have pretty much eliminated sugar. I also take a number of dietary supplements. I still try to keep my fat intake to about 25 percent of daily calories and not go overboard on protein.

This new regimen has been great. I have more energy, and there has been a complete change in my moods. I notice that for many of our guests who are sixty and older, cutting down on carbohydrates and using supplements appropriately seem to produce good results.

I never dreamed that Canyon Ranch would evolve into what it is today, a very integrative health and education center. Nutrition reigns supreme here. The knife and fork are powerful tools for improving well-being. You use them three times a day.

2

THE BASICS OF HUMAN NUTRITION

I

THE MACRONUTRIENTS: AN OVERVIEW

Throughout the Western world for at least the past three decades, people have heard that fat is bad for you and have turned to low-fat and nonfat versions of prepared foods. Food manufacturers have learned that the words *low fat* and *nonfat* on labels sell their products. Doctors, nurses, nutritionists, and dietitians all advise cutting fat intake to reduce risks of heart disease and cancer, to lose weight, and to live longer. High-fat foods like butter, cheese, fatty meats and fish, nuts, avocados, and rich desserts are now on the "No" list, because of their perceived ill effects on health and longevity. But as might be expected, their very forbidden nature increases their attractiveness for many.

At the same time, increasing numbers of people have fallen under the spell of a quite different message about diet and health: that carbohydrates, not fat, are the root of all evil, the cause of obesity, high blood pressure, heart disease, deficiency of energy, and feeling low. Low-carbohydrate diets based on this idea, some of which encourage people to eat all the meat, butter, cream, and cheese they want, have become very popular, and their promoters' books are perennial best-sellers.

The Atkins diet, developed by New York cardiologist Robert Atkins, M.D., over twenty-five years ago and now enjoying a resurgence, is the best-known version in the United States. In Europe, its equivalent is the Montignac diet, the invention of a Frenchman, Michel Montignac, a nonphysician who worked as the personnel director of a pharmaceutical company before he embarked on his current career as a diet guru. When I visited Holland in 1997, *le régime Montignac* was sweeping that country, with special restaurants opening to serve rich, low-carbohydrate meals and innumerable Dutch enthusiasts telling everyone how they had shed pounds and gained energy while eating everything previously denied them on conventional reducing diets. As I write, Montignac fever is sweeping the United Kingdom.

A decade ago, when Montignac first published his ideas, the French medical establishment denounced the diet as "a passport to a heart attack." Atkins has been the target of similar scorn from doctors in America, especially from those who advocate extremely low fat diets. The Pritikin Institute, brainchild of the late entrepreneur Nathan Pritikin, puts people with high blood pressure, heart disease, adult-onset diabetes, and other chronic diseases on diets with no more than 10 percent of total calories as fat and gets many good results. Pritikin meals emphasize grains (including bread and pasta), vegetables, fruits, and moderate amounts of low-fat preparations of fish and chicken. The institute teaches that fat is the root of all evil, and that the ideas of Atkins and Montignac are dangerous.

Dean Ornish, M.D., the California cardiologist who has demonstrated reversal of coronary heart disease on a program of very low fat vegetarian food, stress reduction, and group support, calls Dr. Atkins "irresponsible." "It's a great way to sell books to tell people that steaks and eggs are health foods, but they're not," he says. He further contends, as do conventional dietitians, that most of the weight loss on a low-carbohydrate, high-fat diet is water, due to a diuretic effect of altered metabolism. "That's ridiculous," Atkins retorts. "When obese patients lose a hundred or more pounds on the Atkins diet, as many do, you're going to tell me that's water? I'm glad Dr. Ornish makes that statement, because it will encourage people to question his credibility."

Such is the contentiousness that divides the camps, and since both sides can cite published studies supporting their positions, it is not easy for people to decide between them. Moreover, there are other positions to consider, such as the recent diet phenomenon called "The Zone." The invention of biochemist Barry Sears, Ph.D., the

Zone diet is a modified Atkins regime with attention paid to kinds of fats and kinds of carbohydrates. Sears urges his many followers to use food as a drug to affect hormones regulating metabolism. He argues that there are good fats and bad fats, in sharp contrast to the "fat is fat" position of the medical mainstream, and he also tries to distinguish between better and worse carbohydrates, separating himself from those who issue blanket denunciations of all sugars and starches. You can "enter the Zone" by eating apples and black beans, but have carrots or pasta and you'll fall out of it into metabolic hellfire and damnation.

So what is it to be: a life with no butter, cheese, oil, and meat, or one with no sugar, bread, potatoes, and pasta? a "plant-based" diet that minimizes or avoids consumption of meat and animal products, or a carnivorous free-for-all that protects health by focusing on the right fats and the right carbohydrates?

Fats and carbohydrates are two of three categories of macronutrients (i.e., "big foods") that our bodies need. The third is protein. These large groupings of foods supply all of the body's caloric or energy needs; in addition, protein provides structural elements for growth and repair of tissue. The body also needs other substances to function normally but in much smaller amounts: vitamins and minerals, for example, and a variety of protective compounds in plants that bolster the body's defenses against the many hazards of living. The term *micronutrients* ("little foods") refers to all those latter elements of diet. In this section I want to explain what we know about macronutrients from scientific research with a view toward specifying their place in the optimum diet.

I will examine the roles of fats, carbohydrates, and proteins in human health and nutrition to see if there are answers to the kinds of disagreements I have sketched above, and whether decisions about the macronutrients can be reconciled with the seven principles of diet and health I've already discussed. There are very important questions about how much and what kinds of the big foods we should eat to maintain optimum health, and, although the scientific data is not conclusive, indications are that many prevailing ideas of conventional nutritionists are wrong. In fact, many readers may be surprised by what I have to say, because I believe that some conventional ideas have influenced both popular and medical thinking for the worse, and have spawned styles of cuisine and food preparation that may not be good for us. Obviously, we still have much to learn about human nutrition and the influence of diet on health; neither doctors nor dietitians have all the answers, and on some questions, the experts disagree sharply. I am not afraid to speculate or to try to make good guesses as I venture into unknown territory, but I will always base my speculations on the best available scientific evidence as well as common sense.

Many patients who ask doctors what they should eat to reduce disease risks or treat existing ailments are told, "It doesn't matter; just eat a balanced diet." The general public is well aware that most doctors are essentially uneducated about nutrition. Medical educators object when critics confront them with that fact, pointing out that first-year students receive intensive instruction in biochemistry. But while it is true that nutritional science starts with knowledge of basic biochemistry, it is also true that knowing biochemistry is in no way equivalent to understanding nutrition, let alone to knowing what an optimum diet is or how to advise patients about making dietary changes to improve health.

In order to write about macronutrients, I reviewed a weighty biochemistry text currently being used in medical schools. Biochemistry is a daunting subject, the biggest hurdle first-year medical students have to jump, since it involves rote memorization of the complex details of a great many chemical reactions that take place in living organisms. Students promptly forget these details once their exams are over. It is amusing to ask doctors how many times they learned the Krebs cycle, only to forget it completely. The Krebs cycle, named for German biochemist and later Oxford professor Sir Hans Adolf Krebs, is the central hub of metabolic reactions that generate most of the energy derived from food. I know hardly any physicians who remember the correct sequence of conversions it comprises. Yet the teaching of biochemistry that produces this result often passes for nutritional instruction in medical schools.

Biochemistry provides a scientific basis for understanding why "essential" fatty acids—i.e., those the body needs but cannot make and therefore must be supplied by diet—are necessary, but if that information is buried in a mass of confusing and irrelevant detail, medical students are going to forget it just as quickly as they forget the Krebs cycle once they pass their tests. They are not going to be able to use it in attending to their own diets or advising patients how to improve theirs.

Recently, I asked a class of second-year medical students, their first-year biochemistry experience under their belts, what they knew of one group of essential fatty acids, the omega-3s. These are the unusual fatty acids found in a limited number of foods: mainly oily, cold-water fish and a few seeds and nuts. The students remembered hearing about omega-3 fatty acids in biochemistry, and a few thought they remembered their chemical structure, but none could tell me their nutritional significance or health benefits. In fact, these fats remain fluid at low temperatures and give vital flexibility to cell membranes. (If cold-water fish were insulated with the saturated fat of land animals, they would be stiff as boards and unable to swim.) They are also the compounds from which the body makes hormones that keep blood from clotting abnormally and inflammation from getting out of hand.

The absolute requirement of omega-3s in sufficient daily amounts for good nutrition should be a great concern of doctors who advocate very low fat diets. Most people in Western, industrialized countries are already eating diets deficient in essential fatty acids in general and omega-3 fatty acids in particular. If they now avoid fatty foods in the belief that dietary fat is the chief cause of obesity and illness, this deficiency is likely to become even greater. Ornish, who only recently began recommending that people take supplemental capsules of oils containing omega-3 fatty acids, has said: "You might say, well, why not eat fish, because then you can get the fish oil directly from the fish. And you can. The problem is that the fish that are the highest in the omega-3 fatty acids—salmon and other deep-water fish—are also the highest in fat and cholesterol."

This is a problem only if you consider all fat bad. Salmon is a delicious fish, and its natural oiliness lends it to preparation without added fat, as by steaming, poaching, broiling, or grilling. If you urge people to avoid salmon because of its natural fat content, you encourage them to shun an excellent source of vital nutrients that are hard to find elsewhere. Many doctors who once learned about essential fatty acids to pass biochemistry exams now have no working knowledge of them, and so do not see this danger of the very low fat diets that are popular at spas, clinics, and cardiac rehabilitation centers.

Biochemistry instruction also does not often include, or fails to place proper emphasis on, information of great nutritional significance. For years dietitians have taught people to distinguish between simple carbohydrates (sugars) and complex carbohydrates (starches) and to moderate consumption of the former while increasing intake of the latter. Physicians often pass this information on to patients, but it turns out to be a meaningless distinction and bad advice. What counts, as I will explain in more detail shortly, is how fast a particular carbohydrate food turns into glucose and raises levels of blood sugar, a characteristic expressed numerically as the glycemic index (GI). In general, high-glycemic-index foods stress the pancreas and, in many people, promote weight gain and unhealthy distribution of fats in the blood and tissues. Some complex carbohydrates—potatoes, for instance—have a higher glycemic index and thus raise blood sugar faster than some simple ones like table sugar; such differences influence the short- and long-term effects of these foods on our energy and health. But the biochemistry text I read barely mentioned glycemic index, so it is not surprising that most physicians are unfamiliar with the concept, let alone with how to use it when counseling patients about diet in general and carbohydrate foods in particular.

Here are the big questions I have about the big foods:

- What are the proportions of fat, carbohydrate, and protein in an ideal diet?
- Should you change these proportions if you want to lose or gain weight?
- Are there better and worse carbohydrates? Which carbohydrate foods should predominate in an ideal diet?
- Are there better and worse fats? What are the proportions of different kinds of fat in an ideal diet?
- Are there better and worse sources of protein? What protein foods should predominate in an ideal diet?

In order to answer these questions, I would like to help you understand how the body uses carbohydrate, fat, and protein—how it derives energy from them, stores them, and interconverts them, one into another. In this discussion, I will try not to burden you with more than the mininum amount of biochemical detail necessary to understand the roles of the macronutrients in maintaining life and health.

I wrote earlier that all nutritional energy—what we measure as calories—originates as solar energy that has been captured and stored by green plants. Plants accomplish this feat through photosynthesis, using the energy of light from the red and blue ends of the spectrum* to bind carbon dioxide from the atmosphere and water from the earth into molecules of glucose, releasing oxygen in the process. Glucose, also called dextrose, grape sugar (in plants), and blood sugar (in animals), is one of the simplest carbohydrates, and the most basic food for cells of both plants and animals. It is the fuel many cells prefer to use in order to obtain energy.

When the sun goes down, photosynthesis stops in plants, and the cellular machinery focuses on reversing those reactions. In the reverse process, called respiration, cells "burn" or metabolize newly minted glucose by combining it with oxygen to break the molecule down to carbon dioxide and water and capture the energy that was stored in its chemical bonds. You can burn pure, crystalline glucose in a test tube and watch it give off heat and light. Cellular respiration is a multistep process of controlled burning, the last steps being the famous and forgettable Krebs cycle that generates usable energy in the form of a simple compound called ATP (adenosine triphosphate). ATP is the metabolic currency of all cells, holding most of its energy in the chemical bond linking the phosphate group to the rest of the molecule.

Not long ago, nurses in hospitals performed a superstitious ritual at dusk. They went from room to room removing flowers and plants from patients' bedsides in the belief that living plants robbed oxygen from the air at night. In fact, plants, like animals, are always respiring at the cellular level, always using oxygen, both day and night, to obtain their energy needs. The amount of oxygen a bouquet of flowers or even a potted plant removes during the night is insignificant compared to that used by the person sleeping in the next bed. But the oxygen released by an actively photosynthesizing plant is significant,

---

*Green plants appear green to us because they reflect back light from the unused middle portion of the visible light spectrum.

and the total amount released into the atmosphere by the green bio-mass of the planet makes it possible for animals to live. So there is a wonderful interdependence of these two biological kingdoms: Both plants and animals take in oxygen and release carbon dioxide all the time as they burn stored energy, but, in addition, green plants exposed to light use the waste carbon dioxide from animals as a starting material for making glucose, releasing oxygen in the process. And, of course, animals eat plants (and plant-eating animals) to get the solar energy they cannot capture directly.

Active tissues of both plants and animals (growing shoots and leaves, the brain) need large, constant amounts of glucose and have elaborate hormonal controls to regulate the distribution and fate of this simple sugar and its content of solar energy. The metabolism of glucose is disturbed in obesity and in diabetes, though which is cause and which is effect is not clear. If blood glucose drops too low (as can happen if a person with diabetes injects too much insulin or eats too little), fatigue and weakness develop rapidly, followed by unconsciousness, symptoms that disappear in seconds following an intravenous injection of a glucose solution. The brain is just that dependent on a constant, steady supply of glucose. It also requires a disproportionate share of the body's total metabolic energy, and so is a major consumer of glucose in the blood.

CARBOHYDRATES

Carbohydrates are compounds made up of carbon, hydrogen, and oxygen, arranged in ring structures that can be linked together end to end to form more complex molecules. The simplest carbohydrates are single-ring sugars: glucose, fructose (fruit sugar), and galactose (a milk sugar), collectively called monosaccharides, meaning sugars composed of one ring. Two of these rings linked together make disaccharides, such as maltose (glucose plus glucose), produced by sprouting grains and abundant in beer. Sugar-cane plants and sugar beets make quantities of another, very familiar disaccharide called sucrose or table sugar (glucose plus fructose). Lactose, the main sugar in milk, is also a disaccharide (glucose plus galactose).

You may know people who are lactose intolerant. They lack a digestive enzyme needed to split this disaccharide into its monosaccharide components for metabolic processing. If these people drink milk, they suffer digestive upsets: belching, rumbling, and flatulence, the result of bacterial digestion of milk sugar in the gut with abundant production of methane gas. A similar inability to break down more complex sugars that occur in beans accounts for the flatulence that often follows eating them. Such indigestible sugars are often called resistant carbohydrates, because they resist digestion by our systems. One class of resistant carbohydrates includes very large molecules that make up structural components of plants; cellulose, for example, gives toughness to plant cell walls. Collectively, these substances are known as fiber, and they have important roles as micronutrients in human nutrition.

Sugars are osmotically active, meaning they draw water molecules toward themselves through porous membranes like those enclosing cells. This property makes it impossible for plants and animals to store energy in the form of sugars. If too much glucose were to accumulate in a cell, the cell would quickly swell and burst. Therefore, to store energy, organisms must convert the glucose they make into something else. Plants often turn sugars into starches, much larger carbohydrate molecules of different chemical structure that do not draw water across cell membranes and so are convenient for storing energy for later use. The most common storage sites for starch are roots (sweet potatoes), underground stems (white potatoes), fruits (winter squashes), and seeds (beans and grains). There are two principal plant starches, amylose and amylopectin. Amylose consists of long chains of glucose rings strung together like single, tight strands of beads. In amylopectin, the chains have many side branches.

When we eat starchy vegetables, fruits, and grains, our bodies turn these complex carbohydrates back into glucose for metabolic fuel, but the different structural characteristics of amylose and amylopectin affect the speed of this conversion, amylopectin being much easier to digest because its branches offer more surfaces for enzymes to work on. This difference is important because it is a major determinant of glycemic index—of how fast various starchy foods affect our blood sugar levels, which, in turn, affects our energy, our tendency to gain weight, and our general health. The main form of starch in the sticky, white rice that Japanese and Chinese people steam and eat as a staple carbohydrate with most meals is amylopectin. Steamed white basmati rice, a staple grain of India, looks and tastes quite different, with drier, separate grains, because its starch is mostly amylose. "Diet gurus" who warn people away from white rice as a refined carbohydrate that wreaks havoc with blood sugar ignore this difference. Even if you are "carbohydrate sensitive," you can enjoy some white rice if you choose a lower-glycemic-index variety like basmati.

Animals can turn glucose into their own form of starch, called glycogen, and store it in the liver and muscles as a short-term energy reserve. Glycogen, like amylopectin, is highly branched, making for rapid conversion to glucose. If you stop eating (or stop eating carbohydrates) you have enough glycogen in the liver to maintain blood glucose for about forty-eight hours if you are sedentary, less if you are active. Exercise vigorously and your glycogen supply will run out quickly. After it does, your body will have to find another source of glucose for metabolic fuel. Endurance athletes, like marathon runners, know this point well and call it "hitting the wall." It represents the lag time between using up the last of the glycogen and shifting metabolism into another mode to burn protein and fat instead. Athletes say it feels like an overwhelming drop in available energy, and to gain time before it happens, they often indulge in "carbohydrate loading" before events—eating large quantities of pasta, for example, in order to maximize glycogen stores.

FATS

Plants and animals can condense energy further by turning glucose into fats for even longer-term storage. Fats are mixtures of fatty acids, chains of carbon atoms linked together, most of them attached to hydrogen atoms, with a distinctive oxygen-containing group at one end of the chain—the weakly acid end. The carbon-carbon bonds in fatty acids are more energetic than those in carbohydrates; as a result fats have almost twice the calories of carbohydrates, gram for gram.

Oils are liquid fats. The term *lipids* includes all of these substances: fats, oils, their constituent fatty acids, and more complex compounds built from them. Plants often store oils in seeds (nuts, sesame seeds, corn), only rarely in fruits (olives, avocados), and almost never in any quantity elsewhere. Their purpose in seeds is to provide concentrated energy for the growing embryo of the next generation. We store fat under the skin in all the familiar places as energy reserves in anticipation of hard times, as well as to insulate the body and cushion vital organs. We also make fat easily from glucose, so that any food that can be broken down to glucose can also be converted to fat. When caloric intake exceeds expenditures, the body will store the excess of fat. Conversely, whenever caloric expenditures exceed intake and liver and muscle glycogen is exhausted, fat reserves are mobilized for metabolism.

Stored fat cannot be converted to energy as quickly or as easily as glycogen can, one reason for the phenomenon of "hitting the wall." To obtain energy from fat, the body breaks down fatty acid molecules into two-carbon fragments ("acetate fragments") that cells can burn in their metabolic furnaces, combining them with oxygen and producing carbon dioxide and water as waste products. Most, but not all, cells can carry out this process, called fatty acid oxidation. Muscle is particularly good at it, so when muscle cells run out of glycogen, they begin getting energy from fatty acids. During prolonged fasting, most tissues use fatty acids as fuel, but some cannot. Brain cells, in particular, cannot get their energy needs from fatty acids. They can, however, burn some of the intermediate breakdown products of fatty acids that the liver releases into the bloodstream when it burns fats. These molecules, called ketone bodies, become important during starvation, when they build up to sufficient levels in the blood for the brain to take them in and use them as an alternative energy source—a situation called ketosis.

Remember that the highly specialized cells of the brain prefer to run on glucose, the simplest fuel. But an important fact of human nutrition is that, although our bodies can easily turn glucose into fat, they cannot turn fat back into glucose. This basic biochemical limitation has profound implications for people who are starving and for dieters who restrict or eliminate intake of carbohydrates. Physicians have noted that people experiencing ketosis, when the brain is denied a source of glucose and is forced to burn ketone bodies, often report feelings of well-being and the absence of hunger. Dr. Atkins and his imitators suggest that the same situation obtains on their low-carbohydrate diets, that people following them go into ketosis and experience decreased hunger and increased mental and physical energy as a result.

It is not clear that this is the case, because the popular low-carbohydrate diets are very high in protein, and, as I will explain shortly, the body can make glucose from protein when it is deprived of its usual sources. I think the brain can still get its usual fuel on an Atkins/Montignac regime, but I am concerned that its method of doing so may have long-term detrimental effects on health.

Fatty acids come in three varieties. In saturated fatty acids (SFAs) all available carbon bonds are occupied by—or saturated with—hydrogen atoms. These are the fat molecules the body prefers to break down to acetate fragments and burn for energy, so it is not surprising that stored animal fat is mostly composed of SFAs. (Remember those acetate fragments. I will return to them later when I discuss cholesterol, because the body uses them as starting materials to make that substance. They are the all-important link between diet and cardiovascular disease.) Monounsaturated fatty acids (MUFAs) have one link in the chain where two carbon atoms share two bonds with each other instead of one. This double bond is a point of strain in the fatty acid chain that affects its shape and chemical nature. MUFAs occur in the oils of many nuts and seeds and also dominate the fatty acid profiles of olive oil and avocados. Our body fat contains MUFAs, too, and the body can burn them for energy.

Polyunsaturated fatty acids (PUFAs) have two or more double bonds, and predominate in the oils obtained from the seeds of safflowers, sunflowers, sesame, corn, and soy. The body can convert some of these into SFAs for fuel, but it has special uses for PUFAs that are important to understand. It incorporates them into membranes of cells and intracellular organelles (i.e., the "little organs" like mitochondria and ribosomes that exist within cells), taking advantage of their flexibility and water-repelling property to hold and protect the watery contents of these structures. The body also synthesizes important hormones from PUFAs, including steroid hormones and prostaglandins.

All fats and oils are mixtures of fatty acids, and the percentages of the three varieties of constituent fatty acids can be specified. For example, olive oil contains 14 percent SFAs, 77 percent MUFAs, and 9 percent PUFAs, and so is classified as a monounsaturated oil. In beef fat the percentages are 51 for SFAs, 44 for MUFAs, and 5 for PUFAs, making it a predominately saturated fat. Saturated fats tend to be solid at room temperature. Polyunsaturated vegetable oils remain liquid at low temperatures, and MUFAs are in between. I will have more to say about dietary fats and lipid metabolism because they have important influences on health and longevity.

PROTEINS

To make the third kind of macronutrient—proteins—plants combine simple sugars with nitrogen from the air or soil to make amino acids, the building blocks of these compounds. Proteins are much larger and much more complex than carbohydrates and fats, with intricate, distinctive three-dimensional shapes, and each organism has unique proteins that establish its biological identity in addition to others that are common among many forms of life. (In deciding whether substances it encounters belong in the body or not, the immune system mostly pays attention to protein chemistry; it is the unique proteins of an organism that determine what is "self" and what is "not-self.") Protein makes up most of the weight of the human body that is not water.

Animals break down the proteins they eat into their constituent amino acids, then rearrange those building blocks into the protein molecules they need for growth and repair. They can also synthesize many amino acids, but not all. For humans, ten amino acids are "essential," meaning they must be supplied by the diet in order for the body to manufacture the proteins it needs. Without them, protein deficiency and malnutrition result quickly because the body cannot store nitrogen or amino acids in the way it can store carbohydrates and fat.

You can think of amino acids—there are twenty of them that make up all animal proteins—as the letters that spell out a great variety and number of different protein "words." Cells contain tiny protein factories (ribosomes) that receive coded instructions from DNA in the cell nucleus for putting amino acids together into long chains. Once complete, these chains assume complicated coiled and twisted structures determined by the chemical and electrical characteristics and sequence of their amino acid subunits. The usefulness of proteins in the body depends on these distinctive three-dimensional shapes. For example, actin and myosin, the proteins that compose muscle fibers, have unique shapes that allow them to slide over one another in response to signals from nerves, resulting in muscle contraction. Collagen and elastin give skin its remarkable qualities of toughness and flexibility.

Another important category of proteins is enzymes. The alchemy by which both plants and animals transform the basic product of photosynthesis, glucose, into a range of sugars, starches, fats, and proteins depends on enzymes, specialized protein molecules that control biochemical reactions. Enzymes can turn sugars into starches, starches into glucose, sugars into fats, fats into acetate fragments for fuel, acetate fragments into cholesterol, sugars into proteins, and proteins back into sugars, depending on the organism's needs. Many of these conversions are the same in plants and animals, the main differences being that plants can make glucose from carbon dioxide, water, and sunlight and can make amino acids and proteins from scratch, using nitrogen from the soil. Enzymes are responsible for all of these reactions.

Here is how I described them in my book *Spontaneous Healing*:

Enzymes catalyze the chemical reactions of life—that is, they speed up the rates at which these reactions reach equilibrium but are not themselves changed in the process. Enzymes are necessary because if left to themselves, the reactions would not take place fast enough to support life. Chemists can speed up indolent reactions by subjecting them to high temperatures and pressures and by creating extreme conditions of acidity or alkalinity (pH). They can also add chemical catalysts to reactions, but these, too, often work best under physical conditions far removed from those of cells, which live at relatively low temperatures, at atmospheric pressure, and at nearly neutral pH. By contrast, enzymes in cells are able to catalyze reactions under the mild conditions of life and do so with much greater efficiency than their inorganic counterparts. They may be thought of as highly complex and efficient molecular machines.

How do enzymes work? The answer has to do with their three-dimensional configurations, which give them the ability to bind with great specificity to other molecules—substrates—and accelerate their tendency to react. The binding takes place at a particular site on the enzyme, which is both geometrically and electronically complementary to a portion of the substrate. Many enzymes will bind only to one substrate and not to any other molecule, even a very close relative. Once bound to an enzyme, the substrate may find itself in physical proximity to another reactant or it may be forced into a new configuration that strains particular chemical bonds, making them more likely to break or reform in ways that favor a desired reaction. Enzymes have diverse mechanisms by which they cause chemical bonds of substrates to change. In practical terms, they function as ingenious machines that alter substrate molecules: cutting them apart, putting them together, snipping particular pieces off them, adding others back, all with astonishing precision and speed.

For those with lactose intolerance, the problem is one missing or defective enzyme, lactase. If a body produces lactase that is even slightly off from the normal configuration, it will be unable to bind molecules of milk sugar and catalyze their digestion into the component monosaccharides, glucose and galactose.

One more important category of proteins in the body is receptors. Like enzymes, these are molecules designed to bind other molecules in specific ways, but rather than speeding up biochemical reactions, their function is to carry information between and within cells. Many receptors exist within the lipid membranes that enclose cells. For example, insulin receptors are present on the surfaces of most cells. When the pancreas secretes the hormone insulin into the blood, it binds to insulin receptors, and the change in the conformation of the receptor intiates other changes in the cell that allow glucose to pass into the cell and enter into oxidation reactions to produce energy. Deficiency or loss of insulin receptors is the biochemical correlate of insulin resistance, which in its extreme form is the immediate cause of adult-onset (also called type II and non-insulin-dependent) diabetes. In this disease, the pancreas makes insulin, but cells cannot respond to it; their sensitivity to insulin is diminished. As a result, blood sugar is persistently elevated, and the whole energy economy of the body is deranged.

This is not an exhaustive catalog of uses of protein in the body, but I think it conveys a sense of their key roles in maintaining life. It is also important to know that if the diet supplies more protein than the body needs to build, maintain, and repair itself, the excess goes into the metabolic furnace for fuel. Digestion breaks dietary protein into its consitituent amino acids, and many of the amino acids are easily turned into glucose, which can be burned, turned into glycogen, or converted to fat for storage, depending on energy needs. You must also know that the metabolism of protein as an energy source is quite different from that of fat and carbohydrates because of protein's nitrogen content. Fat and carbohydrates are clean-burning fuels, releasing only carbon dioxide and water as the final by-products of oxidation. Protein, in addition, leaves a residue of ammonia, a simple compound of nitrogen and hydrogen that many of us know as a household cleaning agent or a fertilizer. Ammonia is extremely toxic, especially to brain cells, and its generation in the course of oxidizing amino acid fuels creates a major problem of elimination for the body. I will write more about this and its relevance to determining how much protein the optimum diet should contain when I return to the subject of protein later in this chapter.

I mentioned earlier that while the body cannot obtain glucose from fat, it can make it from protein. Many amino acids can serve as substrates for the synthesis of glucose in the liver, a process called gluconeogenesis, Greek for "creating glucose from scratch." During starvation, the brain's demand for glucose causes the body to sacrifice its own muscle tissue in order to support gluconeogenesis, so that weight loss in starvation represents not only the metabolism of stored fat but also loss of lean body mass. The possibility that this may also happen on low-carbohydrate diets is cause for concern. Even if people on these diets are eating a lot of protein, the absence of dietary carbohydrate may still encourage the body to turn to its own muscle tissue as a source of amino acids for gluconeogenesis to feed the brain.

I have now sketched the basic facts I believe to be relevant to an understanding of the nature of the macronutrients and their roles in human biology. Let me review and summarize them before looking at each category more closely.

Carbohydrates—sugars and starches—are mainly used for energy production through conversion to glucose and its subsequent oxidation. They are readily usable, clean-burning fuels. Glucose can be burned immediately, converted to animal starch—glycogen—for short-term storage in the liver and in muscles, or converted to fatty acids for long-term storage. The body can adapt to a wide range of carbohydrate intake, but too much over time will cause most people to store too much fat, while too little can precipitate ketosis, an alternative pathway of energy production that may be detrimental to long-term health. All tissues of the body can use glucose as fuel, many prefer it, and some, notably the brain, use it exclusively except in unusual circumstances (such as starvation). Different carbohydrate foods are more or less quickly digested and converted to glucose (a reflection of the glycemic index), requiring the pancreas to produce more or less insulin to deal with the rate of increase of glucose in the blood. In both diabetes and obesity, carbohydrate metabolism is disturbed.

Fats and oils are long-term energy reserves, made up of fatty acids, molecules that hold more energy than carbohydrates, are equally clean-burning, but are not so readily usable. In addition to providing a storage form of energy, lipids compose cell membranes and serve as substrates for the synthesis of hormones. Fatty acids occur in saturated (SFAs), monounsaturated (MUFAs), and polyunsaturated (PUFAs) forms, and which category predominates in a given fat or oil determines its physical and chemical characteristics. The body burns SFAs and MUFAs as fuels, but uses PUFAs as membrane components and hormone substrates. Some PUFAs are essential; the diet must provide them or illness will result.

Many cells can use fatty acids as energy sources, but some (brain cells) cannot; the latter can use intermediate breakdown products of fatty acid oxidation (ketone bodies) produced by the liver when carbohydrates are not available. Although the body easily turns glucose into fatty acids, it cannot reverse the process and make glucose from fatty acids. Excess consumption of fat leads, in most people, to excess storage of body fat and excess circulation of lipids in the blood, both of which can be detrimental to health. (Dietary fat is converted to stored body fat more efficiently than dietary carbohydrate is converted to stored body fat.) Insufficient consumption of fat increases the risk of essential fatty acid deficiency, with many attendant consequences for health.

Protein, unlike carbohydrates and fat, contains nitrogen in addition to carbon, hydrogen, and oxygen. Protein molecules are made up of chains of amino acids that assume specific three-dimensional configurations; these shapes determine their functions. The body needs regular intake of proteins in order to build, maintain, and repair itself. Protein makes up much of the structure of the body, including muscles and skin, as well as much of its regulatory apparatus (enzymes, receptors). All proteins in the body are built from a pool of twenty different amino acids, ten of which are essential and must be supplied by the diet on an ongoing basis, since the body cannot store free amino acids or nitrogen. The body can make the ten nonessential amino acids starting from glucose, and it can derive glucose from a number of amino acids.

If the diet contains more protein than the body needs to build, maintain, and repair itself, it will use the excess as fuel, but protein is not a clean-burning fuel, because the nitrogen-containing residue it leaves in the form of ammonia is toxic and must be eliminated. When deprived of carbohydrate sources of glucose, the liver can manufacture glucose from protein (gluconeogenesis), often using muscle tissue as a source. Excess consumption of protein may increase the workload of the digestive system and places a particular burden on the liver and kidneys. Insufficient consumption of protein is a common cause of malnutrition, wasting, increased susceptibility to disease, and early death in many underdeveloped countries.

That concludes an overview of the macronutrients. I would now like to look at each category more closely to explain its place in the optimum diet.

II

CARBOHYDRATES REVISITED: STAFF OF LIFE OR STUFF OF SICKNESS?

A popular brand of cornstarch sold in America uses as its logo the image of an Indian maiden whose body is an ear of golden corn. She has been known to several generations of American housewives, and has been even better known to countless earlier generations of Native Americans, for she is the corn goddess, personifying the spirit of the plant that has helped sustain human life in the New World. Corn (maize) is unique among cereal grains in that it is wholly dependent on human intervention for its own survival. The husks that envelop an ear of corn prevent the individual grains from germinating. Corn is thus a human invention, the product of complex interbreeding of ancestral grains, greatly modified by human selection.

Like other grains, maize seeds contain carbohydrate, protein, and fat. The largest fraction of their total caloric content is starch that the germinating seed can convert to glucose and burn to get the energy needed for initial growth, until it produces enough young leaf to photosynthesize its own food. That Native Americans deified this plant is a statement of its importance in their world. Throughout history in the Americas, an abundant maize harvest meant health, happiness, and assurance of food through the winter; crop failure meant starvation and untimely death.

In other parts of the world people held other cereal grains in equally high esteem because they depended on them in the same way for health and life. In Japan rice planting was, and still is, for many, a religious act, in which people invoke the aid of Ta No Kami, the Shinto god of rice paddies, to protect the plants and assure a good harvest. Tibetans are as reverent about the cultivation of barley, a grain that can be adapted to short-season areas.

These crops are usually called dietary staples because they are the most basic elements of human nutrition, and products made from them, which provide most calories in the form of starch, often help define cultural identity. Think of the rice bowl in Asia, tortillas in Mexico, rye bread in northern Europe, and wheat bread in the rest of Europe and most of North America. I once spent time in Ethiopia, where I ate *wat*, grayish sheets of a unique, spongy bread made from an indigenous staple grain called teff, with every meal. I learned to sop up spicy stews and gravies with this staple carbohydrate food that is the signature of Ethiopian cuisine. In other cultures, the starchy staples are roots and tubers rather than seeds. Andean Indians eat more than eighty varieties of potatoes in a dazzling array of shapes and colors, and Amazonian Indians depend on yuca, one product of which is tapioca. But whether seeds or tubers, all of these staples are sources of starch—carbohydrate—with or without accompanying protein and fat.

In our own culture, bread, usually made from refined wheat flour, is served with most meals. I suspect that our ancestors, rather than politely eating rolls with butter while waiting for first courses to arrive, tore hunks of bread off large loaves and used them to sop up sauces, gravies, and juices, much as Ethiopians do with their *wat*. In lean times, there might have been nothing to sop; many meals might have consisted of bread alone. Bread has earned the designation "staff of life" because people in our culture have long been supported by it. It has often stood between them and hunger.

But people cannot have leaned on this staff forever, because bread is a relatively recent invention in the history of the human race, dating back only to the domestication of wheat, about nine thousand years ago, in the Fertile Crescent of the Middle East. This raises the question of what people depended on for their basic supply of calories before the development of agriculture and the cultivation of cereals.

In recent years, a number of medical experts have conjectured about human nutrition in truly ancient times—as far back as the Stone Age, well before the invention of agriculture. In writing about the Paleolithic diet of our distant ancestors, they claim that it was superior to contemporary habits of eating. I always read these articles with interest and, later in this book, will consider the Paleolithic diet as a contender for the optimum diet.

But I detect a certain romanticism in accounts of the Paleolithic diet. Our hunter-gatherer ancestors come across as being happier and healthier than us, with much more leisure time, and none of the social inequalities and stresses of modern urbanites. Of course, day-to-day reality in the Stone Age was probably not so rosy. Death from violence, accident, and infection must have been very common. Few individuals lived beyond what is now considered youth, so most did not live long enough to develop the degenerative diseases that are common in our times and are often blamed on our eating habits.

Remnants of these Stone Age societies persist in our world—in Amazonia, in the deserts of southern Africa, in the rain forests of Papua New Guinea, and in a few other locations. Recently, I made the brief acquaintance of a few of these people, members of a dwindling band of bushmen, refugees who had reluctantly sought help from a game reserve that I visited in Namibia in southern Africa. I spent a morning following them through desert scrub as they demonstrated their methods of hunting with spears and foraging for occasional edible tubers at the bases of dessicated shrubs. It did not look to me like an easy method of obtaining food, but anthropologists consistently report that successful hunter-gatherer societies do, in fact, have much more leisure time than we do and are well nourished.

Their nourishment consists primarily of wild game (animals, birds) and fish, supplemented by inconstant additions of wild fruits, nuts, and starchy tubers. Probably the most significant difference from our way of eating is that none of this food is refined or processed. Another is the relative absence of carbohydrate.

Rhapsodic praise for the Paleolithic diet by anthropologists and some physicians resonates with the anticarbohydrate advocates. We are told that the advent of agriculture and the introduction of cereal grains in the human diet started us on the road to obesity, diabetes, atherosclerosis, and all manner of ills of modern civilization, social as well as physical.*

The reasoning behind this assertion goes like this: Cultivation of grains and secondarily of starchy tubers and roots introduced large amounts of carbohydrate into the human diet on a regular basis. Prior to that development, early humans got sugar only occasionally in the form of wild fruit or honeycombs and starch only occasionally in the form of wild nuts and tubers. This change required the pancreas to work much harder, because insulin is needed to manage the flood of glucose into the bloodstream that follows every high-carbohydrate meal. High levels of blood glucose (hyperglycemia) are toxic and must be cleared rapidly to maintain normal body function. One problem they create is abnormal reactions of glucose with protein molecules (glycation) that can result in defective enzymes and tissues. Glycation may account for some of the degenerative changes commonly seen in people with diabetes, such as vascular and retinal damage.

Like all hormones, insulin has widespread and varied effects in the body even though doctors typically pay attention to only one of them: the facilitation of transport of glucose from the blood into cells. We now know that insulin also encourages the body to store up calories as fat, can promote arterial damage, and may even accelerate the growth of tumors. Moreover, in some people, frequent outbursts of insulin from the pancreas may encourage cells to decrease their sensitivity to that hormone. By making fewer insulin receptors, they become insulin resistant. Insulin resistance is associated with stubborn obesity, abnormalities of blood fats, high blood pressure, adult-onset diabetes, and cardiovascular disease, including increased risk of death from heart attacks and strokes. Is it possible that all those satisfying, filling, life-sustaining carbohydrate foods that became available to us following the domestication of starch-bearing plants are the root cause of these calamities?

One tool for analyzing this question is the glycemic index (GI), the measure of how different carbohydrate foods affect blood glucose. The higher the GI, the faster is the rate of increase of glucose in the

---

*The invention of agriculture is blamed by various experts for urbanization and its attendant evils (overcrowding, pollution, crime), gender inequality, maldistribution of wealth, and dwindling leisure time.

blood, the greater the insulin response, and the greater the potential to expose the body both to the toxic effects of high blood sugar and to the harmful effects of insulin. Glycemic index is a relatively new concept, one that has gained recent acceptance among nutritionists and physicians in Europe but has not made much headway in America, where outmoded and less useful ways of viewing carbohydrates are still in vogue.

To measure glycemic index, researchers feed measured portions of a carbohydrate food to a panel of volunteers who then give blood samples at regular intervals for determination of glucose levels. Here is how one scientist doing this work describes the process:

1. An amount of food containing 50 grams of carbohydrate is given to a volunteer to eat. For example, to test boiled spaghetti, the volunteer would be given 200 grams of spaghetti, which supplies 50 grams of carbohydrate (we work this out from food composition tables). Fifty grams of carbohydrate is equivalent to 3 tablespoons of pure glucose powder.

2. Over the next two hours . . . we take a sample of their blood every 15 minutes during the first hour and thereafter every 30 minutes. The blood sugar level of these blood samples is measured in the laboratory and recorded.

3. The blood sugar level is plotted on a graph and the area under the curve is calculated using a computer program.

4. The volunteer's response to spaghetti (or whatever food is being tested) is compared with his or her blood sugar response to 50 grams of pure glucose (the reference food).

5. The reference food is tested on two to three separate occasions and an average value is calculated. This is done to reduce the effect of day-to-day variation in blood sugar responses.

6. The average GI found in 8 to 10 people is the GI of that food.

Glucose is assigned an arbitrary GI of 100. All other carbohydrates have a GI of less than 100 (except for maltose, a disaccharide consisting of two linked glucose molecules, which is rated at 105). Foods with GIs below 55 are considered to have a low glycemic index. Numbers above 70 indicate a high glycemic index, and numbers between 55 and 70 are intermediate. Scientists have now measured the glycemic index for many different carbohydrate foods; sample results are shown in the table on pages 56–7.*

In general, high-glycemic-index foods provoke strong insulin responses, increasing exposure of the body to all the harmful effects of that hormone, whereas low-glycemic-index foods do not. Low-glycemic-index foods provide energy in slow- and sustained-release form, mitigating hunger and facilitating the smooth use and storage of calories. High-glycemic-index foods provide bursts of energy that may be followed quickly by depletions and hunger. This does not necessarily mean that high-GI foods are bad and low-GI foods are good, but it may mean that the proportion of high-GI foods in the diet is an important variable to consider in looking at the health risks of relying on carbohydrates as staples.

Several factors influence how fast a particular carbohydrate raises blood sugar. One is the chemical nature of the carbohydrate. The body is very efficient at processing glucose, its preferred fuel, but it has a limited ability to handle fructose, a common monosaccharide in fruits and honey. Fructose has quite a low GI of 23. Remember that ordinary table sugar, sucrose, is a disaccharide made up of one molecule of glucose linked to one of fructose. The GI of white sugar is 65, almost exactly midway between 23 and 100, in the intermediate range. As I said earlier, amylose and amylopectin, the two principal plant starches, have different rates of digestion. Amylopectin has a higher GI than amylose, because its branched structure gives enzymes more surface area to attack.

Even more important is the physical nature of the carbohydrate in a particular food. Most breads are in the high range, not because of the chemical nature of wheat starch, but for two mechanical reasons. First, the fine particle size of wheat flour gives digestive enzymes great surface area to work on, and second, the exploded structure of bread, a result of the leavening action of yeast, further increases the surface area of the food. By contrast, pasta has a low GI, which can be lowered further by cooking it less. The *al dente* pasta that Italians favor and that seems slightly undercooked to Americans when they

---

*Note that an alternative GI scale using white bread as the reference food appears in some of the nutritional literature. If bread is assigned a GI of 100, then the GI of glucose is 130. If you see values above 100 for foods like potatoes and rice, they come from this alternative scale. I hope we will soon have uniformity in this area. It makes more sense to me to have the GI scale run from 0 to 100 with glucose at the top.

first encounter it resists digestive enzymes more than longer-cooked pasta and so has a lower GI.

If you look over listings of GIs for representative foods, you will probably be surprised. Some foods that have a reputation as being austere, "diet" foods—rice cakes and crispbread, for example—have very high GIs, while many sugary foods rate lower. Rice cakes have a profound impact on blood sugar because the starch is puffed up, offering great surface area for digestion, whereas sugar is low because half of its molecules are fructose, which we do not metabolize well.

Other factors affect glycemic index as well. The presence of fiber is a moderating influence, because fibrous coats around beans and seeds and the cellulose in intact plant cell walls restrict access by digestive enzymes to the starch within. Beans and some grains like oats contain soluble fiber that makes intestinal contents more viscous, slowing down digestion of their starch. The fiber in whole wheat is insoluble. If wheat grains are whole or cracked, this acts as a physical barrier to digestion, but when whole-wheat grains are finely milled, this effect is lost. That is why whole-wheat bread has about the same GI as white bread. There may be advantages to using whole-wheat flour over white flour (it contains more vitamins and minerals, and its insoluble fiber increases intestinal bulk), but moderating the effect of digestion of wheat starch on blood sugar is not one of them.

The presence of fat in a food reduces glycemic index by slowing the rate of emptying of the stomach and so also the digestion of starch. For this reason (along with the presence of sugar) oatmeal cookies have a lower GI than oatmeal. That does not mean they are better for you. This effect of fat is misleading. If you want to modify your carbohydrate intake in order to protect yourself from the harmful effects of high blood sugar and excessive insulin secretion, adding fat to your starchy foods is not the best way to do it. A better strategy is to add acids, such as vinegar, lemon juice, and acidic fruits, because increased gastric acidity also slows stomach emptying and digestion.

I want to explain how this new concept of rating carbohydrate foods by glycemic index makes it possible to understand the impact of those foods on human nutrition historically and at present, as well as to decide how much and what kind of carbohydrate should be in the optimum diet. Before I do, I must tell you how the concept has been misused, distorted, and bastardized by popular writers.

In the first place, people in everyday life do not eat measured portions of single-carbohydrate foods. They eat complex meals, containing foods that provide varying amounts of carbohydrate along with protein, fat, fiber, and other micronutrients. Glycemic index applies only to the carbohydrate portion of a meal, but even if that portion comprises a number of different foods, the GI of a meal can be calculated fairly easily. First, the total grams of carbohydrate in the meal are added up. Then the percentage of that total contributed by each food is determined. Next, that percentage is multiplied by the food's GI. For example, if your breakfast contains 60 grams of carbohydrate and includes two slices of toast (13 grams of carbohydrate each), the toast accounts for 43 percent of the total (26 divided by 60 times 100). Forty-three percent of 70, the GI for bread, equals about 30. By doing the same calculation for the other sources of carbohydrate in the breakfast and adding the figures, the GI of the meal is determined.

I am not recommending that you have GI tables, carbohydrate counters, and a calculator by your plate when you sit down to a meal. The point is that the glycemic index of a meal reflects both the GIs of individual foods making up the meal and their proportional contributions to total carbohydrate. Note that if the only carbohydrate in a meal has a high GI, then the GI of the whole meal is high. For example, if the only carbohydrate in a meal is bread, the GI of that meal is 70. But you can balance the effect on a meal of a high-GI food like bread by including a low-GI food like beans or berries.

Promoters of diets like The Zone and Montignac's ignore this simple fact. They issue blanket condemnations of high-glycemic-index foods, telling people to avoid bread and potatoes, without making them aware of the simple strategy of reducing any harmful effect on blood sugar and insulin response by eating them together with low-glycemic-index foods.

Moreover, these writers fail to point out crucial differences among high-GI foods—for example, that basmati rice and converted rice have lower GIs than Japanese or Chinese steamed rice, or that waxy new potatoes have a lower GI than larger, "floury" potatoes. It is true that ordinary whole-wheat bread and white bread both cause a blood sugar spike, but dense, chewy peasant breads, especially those with

THE GLYCEMIC INDEX OF SOME POPULAR FOODS

KEY

(Glucose = 100)

*Foods containing fat in excess of American Heart Association's guidelines

(av) indicates that the GI is the average of several studies.

GI RANGES The figures form a continuum, but in general:
LOW-GI FOODS .... below 55
INTERMEDIATE-GI FOODS ...... between 55 and 70
HIGH-GI FOODS .... more than 70

BREAKFAST CEREALS

Kellogg's All Bran with extra
    fiber™ 51
Kellogg's Bran Buds with
    Psyllium™ 45
Kellogg's Cocoa Krispies™ 77
Kellogg's Corn Flakes™ 84
Kellogg's Raisin Bran™ 73
Kellogg's Rice Krispies™ 82
Kellogg's Special K™ 54
Oatmeal (old fashioned) 49
Post Shredded Wheat™ 67
Quaker Puffed Wheat™ 67

GRAINS / PASTAS

Buckwheat groats 54
Bulgur 48
Rice
    basmati 58
    brown 55
    long grain, white (av) 56
    short grain, white 72
    Uncle Ben's Converted™ 44
    parboiled 48
Noodles—instant 46
Pasta
    egg fettuccine 32
    ravioli (meat) 39
    spaghetti (av) 43
    spirali 68
Taco shells 68

BREADS, MUFFINS, AND CAKES

Bagel 72
Banana bread* 47
Blueberry muffin* 59
Croissant* 67
Pita bread 57
Pumpernickel (whole grain) 51
Rye bread 76
Sourdough bread 52
Sponge cake 46
Stoneground whole wheat (av) 53
Waffles 76
White bread (av) 70
Whole-wheat bread (av) 69

CRACKERS / CRISPBREAD

Kavli™ 71
Crispbread 81
Ryvita™ 69
Water cracker 78

COOKIES

Arrowroot 69
Graham crackers 74
Oatmeal 55
Shortbread* 64
Social Tea™ biscuits 55
Vanilla wafers 77

VEGETABLES

Beets	69
Carrots	49
Parsnip	97
Peas (green)	48
Potato	
baked (av)	93
new (av)	62
red-skinned	88
French fries	75
Pumpkin	75
Rutabaga	72
Sweet corn	55
Sweet potato	54
Yam	51

LEGUMES

Baked beans (av)	48
Broad beans (av)	79
Butter beans (av)	31
Chickpeas (av)	33
Kidney beans (av)	27
Lentils (av)	30
Navy beans (av)	38
Soy beans (av)	18
Chana dal	8

FRUIT

Apple (av)	38
Apricot (dried)	31
Banana (av)	55
Cantaloupe	65
Cherries	22
Dates, dried	103
Grapefruit	25
Grapes	46
Kiwi	52
Mango	55
Orange (av)	44
Papaya	58
Peach—canned in juice	30
fresh	42
Pear (av)	38
Pineapple	66
Plum	39
Raisins	6
Watermelon	7

DAIRY FOODS

Milk	
whole (av)	22
skim	32
chocolate flavored	34
Ice cream (av)	61
low fat	50
Yogurt, flavored, low fat	33

BEVERAGES

Apple juice	40
Flavored syrup (diluted)	66
Fanta™	68
Gatorade™	78
Orange juice	46

SNACK FOODS

Corn chips*	72
Peanuts	14
Popcorn	55
Potato chips*	54
Pretzels	83

SPORTS BARS

Power Bar™ Performance	
chocolate	58

CANDY

Chocolate*	49
Jelly beans	80
Life Savers™	70
Mars Almond Bar*	68
Twix Cookie Bar™	44
Snickers™	41
Skittles Fruit Chews™	70

SUGARS

Fructose	23
Glucose	100
Honey	58
Lactose	46
Maltose	105
Sucrose	65

some whole or cracked grains, have significantly lower GIs. In their zealous condemnation of starches, Barry Sears, Robert Atkins, and Luc Montignac even lump bread and pasta together in the same category, when scientists have clearly established that pasta has a much lower GI than most bread, one that can be lowered further by preparing it *al dente*.

Some of the recommendations of these writers seem to me to reveal a fundamental misunderstanding of the real-world relevance of glycemic index. They tell people to shun carrots, for example, because carrots have a high GI—as high as 95 in some studies. But remember that to measure glycemic index, volunteers are fed fifty-gram portions of carbohydrate. Carrots contain only about 7 percent carbohydrate, so to get fifty grams of carbohydrate from carrots alone, you would have to eat a *lot* of them. In fact, the test amount was about one and a half pounds. No one ordinarily eats that many carrots at one time, and the amounts that people do eat contribute only moderately to the rise in blood sugar following a mixed meal. Furthermore, carrots are important sources of protective phytochemicals, especially carotenoid pigments that are strong cancer fighters. Telling people to avoid them because of effects on blood sugar is unwise nutritional advice.

Finally, I see a greatly misplaced focus of concern about sugar in the books coming from the low-carbohydrate camp. One of the most popular of those books is called *Sugar Busters* by Leighton Steward. Another is *Sugar Blues* by William Duffy. You should know by now that sugar is no more of a concern than many forms of starch, because starch produces glucose exclusively, whereas sugar (sucrose) yields equal amounts of glucose and the very low GI monosaccharide, fructose.

I have long been fascinated with the antisugar stance of many health food enthusiasts. I have always suspected that part of the reason sugar gets a bad name is just because it is a major source of dietary pleasure. We like sweets; therefore, they must be bad for us. I do not mean to whitewash all the sweet foods in the modern diet or excuse the immoderate consumption of them that is the rule today rather than the exception. A great deal of sugar is added to processed foods to make them taste good, and many of those foods are high in unhealthy fats and high-GI starches and low in micronutrients, not a good recipe for health and longevity. But sugar itself is not the culprit. The problem is more that technology has made so much sugar available and found ways to incorporate it into so many foods that people like.

Human babies come into the world with a strong preference for sweet and a moderate aversion to bitter. All other tastes seem to be learned through a process of social and cultural conditioning. Chinese philosophers identify five basic tastes: sour, bitter, sweet, pungent, and salty, representing the five elements (wood, fire, earth, metal, and water) that compose all things. They say all of these tastes must be present in our food to create nutritional balance, but Americans, like most Westerners, shun bitter.* The Chinese would say this taste avoidance creates the imbalance that impels us to eat too much sweet. (Some bitter flavors you can experiment with to reduce cravings for sweets come from unsweetened coffee and tea, salad greens like radicchio and escarole, some olives, and some cooked greens like chard, mustard, and broccoli rabe.)

In any case, why is a preference for sweet hard-wired into us? Why is the word *sweet* a virtual synonym for *good*? The answer is that sugar is instant energy, requiring less digestive effort to provide glucose to feed the brain, power muscles, and maintain glycogen stores. The liking for sweetness could well be a product of natural selection, since those of our ancestors who had the inclination to seek out ripe fruit and honeycombs, and had the persistence and intelligence to find them, would have been likelier to outrun predators, win fights, and so pass on their genes. If you want to evolve toward living on cosmic energy instead of gross material food, you should probably start by eating more sugar, as that is the food closest to the source.

I should also say that various naturally occurring forms of sugar are essentially the same from the point of view of glycemic index. Eat honey if you like its taste, but it is not better for you than white sugar. (It's actually worse for the teeth, because its stickiness keeps it in contact with dental enamel longer.) It may provide some micronutrients that sugar does not, but it affects blood sugar just about the same. And the various "natural" and "raw" sugars on the market,

*Italians are a notable exception. They eat an array of bitter greens and drink astonishingly bitter aperitifs.

including a new product called "dried cane juice," are as indistinguishable from white sugar in this sense as is finely milled whole-wheat flour from white flour.

Frankly, I am as concerned about flour in the modern diet as I am about sugar. Starch in this finely pulverized form has a higher glycemic index than sugar and occurs in many, many foods, including the breads and pastries that I believe to be major contributors to the epidemic of obesity and cardiovascular disease in modern society.

But this is getting a bit ahead of the story. Let's go back ten thousand years and look at what happened to the human diet when agriculture made starch-bearing plants available on a regular basis. People quickly learned to eat grains, first by parching them, that is, by dry-toasting the whole seeds, then by turning them into gruel and bread (and probably just as early into beer). The human body quickly adapted to these new foods, since it could derive glucose from them so easily, making for better brain function and more energy for physical activity. Human societies thrived as a result, with great increases in population and prosperity.

Think about the sources of carbohydrate in the diet of humans through the millennia following the domestication of crop plants. The list would include whole grains, gruels and porridges made from whole or cracked grains, coarse breads containing cracked and roughly ground grains, beans, vegetables (including tubers and roots), and fruits—all low-GI foods. One nutritional expert writes:

> Food preparation was a simple process: grinding food between stones and cooking it over the heat of an open fire. The result of this process was that all food was digested and absorbed slowly and the usual blood sugar rise was gradual and prolonged. This diet was ideal as far as their bodies were concerned because it provided slow-release energy that helped to delay hunger pangs and provided fuel for working muscles long after the meal was eaten. It was also kind to the pancreas.

Let's consider the sources of carbohydrate in our diets today. Here is a list of the top twenty in the American diet compiled by a researcher at the Harvard School of Public Health:

1.	Potatoes (mashed or baked)	11.	Fruit punch
2.	White bread	12.	Coca-Cola
3.	Cold breakfast cereal	13.	Apple
4.	Dark bread	14.	Skim milk
5.	Orange juice	15.	Pancakes
6.	Banana	16.	Table sugar
7.	White rice	17.	Jam
8.	Pizza	18.	Cranberry juice
9.	Pasta	19.	French fries
10.	Muffins	20.	Candy

I think you will agree that something has changed since 9000 B.C. Experts may quibble about the details of a Mesopotamian brunch, but it is safe to say that our early agriculturalist ancestors were not washing down French fries and pizzas with Coca-Cola and fruit punch. Obviously, people now are getting most of their carbohydrate from high-glycemic-index foods that do not provide slow-release energy and are not at all kind to the pancreas. It is even more interesting that the change happened very recently, mostly in the past two hundred years.

In my view, the problem with carbohydrate in the human diet is not its introduction following the development of agriculture but rather a drastic lowering of the quality of carbohydrate foods as a result of modern food technology, specifically the refining and processing of low-GI foods into high-GI counterparts. Consider two innovations: flour and corn syrup.

Modern flour comes from high-speed rolling mills that replaced traditional millstones in the early 1800s. The new mills were potentially much more efficient, but because they generated much more heat, flour coming from them spoiled more quickly. Spoilage of ground grains results first from rancidity (oxidation) of the oil contained in the embryo of the seed, and oxidation is much accelerated at high temperatures. The solution was to degerminate the grain— that is, remove and discard the embryo—and to remove the seed coat (bran) whose fiber impeded the new milling process. The result was white flour—pure, superfine particles of starch with huge surface area and a very high glycemic index.

Millers could produce this new food much more cheaply than

stone-ground flour, and it had a much longer life in storage. It also turned out to be an easy sell. White flour made lighter, fluffier breads and pastries, and, being a product of new technology, seemed attractively modern. In Europe, city dwellers with sophisticated palates quickly came to prefer these new foods, while the old-fashioned, coarse, dark breads of the past were stigmatized as the fare of peasants and ignorant country-folk.

When I was growing up in mid-twentieth-century America, most bread we ate came in the form of presliced loaves of pure white fluff, so insubstantial that one could easily squeeze a slice to the size of a marble—a popular breakfast table amusement, as I remember. ("Wonder Bread" seemed to me an apt name, indeed.) I still see this stuff in stores, along with a slightly darker version called wholewheat sandwich bread that may have some bran in it for color but compresses just as dramatically and provides starch as equally fine particles for rapid digestion. The bread I am served in most restaurants in North America is not much better, and I am horrified at the successful marketing of this depressing food in Old World countries that should know better. Recently, I traveled through Romania, where most people were eating coarse, dark breads not long ago. I could get nothing but white fluff sliced bread and rolls there, and was told it was possible to find the old-fashioned product only by asking for "health" or "dietetic" bread.

And whether it is shaped into rolls, muffins, or pizza crusts; baked into pretzels or crackers; fortified with vitamins and minerals; or mixed with flours of other grains, these white-flour products are all the same, one of the unhealthiest creations of food technology. Foods made from it are ubiquitous and routinely pull the glycemic index of meals up to levels that cause episodic bursts of high blood sugar (hyperglycemia) and corresponding bursts of insulin secretion (hyperinsulinism).

Corn syrup is a more recent invention, one that has taken the market by storm. Food technologists learned to make a sweet syrup from cornstarch early in this century by boiling it with acid under pressure. The maximum sugar content attained by this method was 42 percent, and the sugar present was mostly glucose. A newer enzyme-mediated process produces corn syrup with higher sugar content, most of it fructose. This product, high-fructose corn syrup, or HFCS, whose sweetness matches that of sucrose, is cheaper than sugar obtained from sugar cane and sugar beets and much loved by manufacturers, who put immense quantities of it into soft drinks, juice, salad dressings, ketchup, jams, jellies, ice cream, and many other foods. Look at labels of sweetened foods, and you will see high-fructose corn syrup everywhere.

I wonder about the metabolic effect of such a great increase in consumption of fructose, which is unprecedented in human history. The Food and Drug Administration (FDA) considers HFCS innocuous, because the body breaks sucrose down into glucose and fructose. In fact, however, the body does not handle large amounts of fructose well. You can maintain life with intravenous glucose, but not with intravenous fructose; severe derangement of liver function results. There is also evidence that high intake of fructose elevates levels of circulating fats (serum triglycerides), increasing risks of disease of the heart and arteries.

In some human populations the disastrous effects of introducing refined and processed carbohydrates are obvious because they happened so rapidly. Two noteworthy examples are native Hawaiians and Native Americans of the desert southwest of the United States. Polynesians are big people who traditionally view stored body fat as a positive attribute, in sharp contrast to the aesthetic of almost anorexic leanness that prevails in Europe and America today. Before contact with Western civilization, the Polynesians who settled the Hawaiian Islands were very active and largely free of the degenerative illnesses that plague them today. Their carbohydrate staples, all with low-glycemic-index ratings, were poi, the mildly fermented paste made from starchy taro roots; breadfruit, high in fiber and micronutrients; and sweet potatoes. They ate meat (pork, especially), fish, shellfish, and other fruits and vegetables. Today they eat a great deal of American fast food, especially bread, rice, soda, snack foods, pastries, and candy. Their normal heaviness has blossomed into morbid obesity accompanied by crippling rates of hypertension, adult-onset diabetes, and heart disease.

In the American Southwest, a similar fate has befallen tribes like the Pimas and O'odham (Papagos), peaceful agriculturalists whose traditional diet of beans, corn, squash, chilies, acorns, and starchy roots has been replaced by the worst offerings of the fast-food and processed-food industries, especially high-GI carbohydrates. These Indians are now hugely fat, with up to 80 percent of the population suffering from adult-onset diabetes. Alarmingly, this disease has begun to appear in children, many of whom become morbidly obese early in grade school. Type II diabetes typically appears in middle age and has not previously been seen in children.

These native peoples are particularly worthy of study because they are close relatives of the Mountain Pima, the only Indians of the region to escape their fate. The Mountain Pima live in remote mountains of the Mexican states of Sonora and Chihuahua and have not yet gained access to modern processed food. They remain lean, active, and free of the diseases of Western civilization, while their relatives from the same gene pool have ballooned into the fat, hypertensive, diabetic Indians who are now so numerous in southern Arizona and northern Mexico.

Even more interesting, when researchers have put some of these Indians back on their traditional foods, the obesity, diabetes, and hypertension have reversed, suggesting that diet is the variable of paramount importance in causing the differences and pointing up the health benefits of unrefined, unprocessed, traditional starchy foods. Similar experiments with native Hawaiians have yielded similar results.

Now why should southwest Indians and Hawaiians be so sensitive to the damaging effects of the modern American diet, especially its emphasis on high-glycemic-index carbohydrates? The likely reason is genetic. Type II diabetes is genetically controlled, but many genes are involved, and its inheritance is not straightforward. Some peoples—Native Americans, gypsies, Eastern European Jews, for example—have these genes in high frequency and often inherit a tendency to this disease, but the examples of the Hawaiians and O'odham tell us that an interplay of genetic and environmental factors is responsible for eliciting type II diabetes. It appears that it is possible to have the genes but not the disease as long as you avoid the environmental triggers. We know that obesity and sedentary lifestyle increase the risks of type II diabetes, presumably only in those people with the genetic susceptibility, and that weight loss and exercise will often cause the disease to recede to the point that no treatment is required. The conventional wisdom is that obesity causes insulin resistance, but might both insulin resistance and obesity be the results of a sensitivity to high-GI carbohydrates?

Carbohydrate sensitivity is a recently popular concept, given more credence by identification of a cluster of symptoms that may act as a marker for it. Called syndrome X or, more accurately, insulin resistance syndrome, and first identified by Gerald Reaven, now a professor emeritus at Stanford University School of Medicine, these symptoms include a tendency to store fat in the abdomen, high blood pressure, and elevated blood fats (serum triglycerides). People with these symptoms, like Hawaiians and O'odham, appear to be very sensitive to the disturbing effects of high-GI carbohydrate foods on metabolism and very prone to develop type II diabetes unless they switch to diets and lifestyles that cause this inherited tendency to recede.

How prevalent is carbohydrate sensitivity? Some experts, like Reaven, estimate that 25 to 30 percent of the general population is very sensitive and more of us are less so. Obviously, if you belong to certain ethnic groups, the risk is higher. Many people do not have this trait, but its prevalence raises another interesting question: Why should a genetic pattern so closely correlated with severe disease be so common in the world? Shouldn't natural selection have weeded such a detrimental trait out of the human gene pool?

An answer that makes sense to me is that the trait has become detrimental only as the environment has changed—specifically, as highly refined and processed carbohydrate foods have become so prominent in human diets in recent years. Before such foods were common, the genes producing carbohydrate sensitivity, insulin resistance, and type II diabetes may actually have been advantageous, especially in populations that did not have regular supplies of calorie-dense foods and that experienced hunger often and starvation sometimes. Some scientists call them "thrifty genes," because they give individuals enhanced ability to take advantage of food when it is available. If you have thrifty genes, you can more easily store up calories as fat, hedging against times when calories are not forthcoming. Thrifty genes become detrimental only when food is available all the time, and, especially, when much of that food is the kind that yields quick-release energy.

If you are carbohydrate-sensitive, what should you do about it? One strategy would be to stop eating carbohydrate foods altogether, and, indeed, this is exactly the recommendation of some of the diet books that are currently so popular. But consider again the studies done with Hawaiians and O'odham. They were not put on a diet of high protein, high fat, and no carbohydrates; they were encouraged to eat their traditional low-GI carbohydrate staples: poi, breadfruit, and sweet potatoes in the former case, and beans, squash, and corn in the latter, and with this change, their metabolic problems reversed. This is an important observation, because it reinforces the idea that it is the kind of carbohydrate you eat that is critical, not whether you eat carbohydrate. Even people genetically programmed for insulin resistance and type II diabetes can be perfectly healthy on diets containing substantial amounts of filling, satisfying, unprocessed, unrefined, low-glycemic-index starchy foods. They may also be able to tolerate moderate amounts of low-GI sweets, especially fruit.

The most facile and pernicious distortion of the scientific evidence by anticarbohydrate writers in popular books about diet, in fitness magazines, and in all manner of publications about health is the suggestion that eating sugar and refined starch is the direct *cause* of insulin resistance and therefore of obesity, diabetes, and cardiovascular disease. This is simply false. Insulin resistance is mostly determined by genetics and strongly influenced by physical fitness and body weight. If you have the genes for it, you can prevent or slow its development by exercising regularly and sufficiently and by keeping weight in the normal range. We are certain to hear a lot more about insulin resistance in the coming years, because it is now an exciting focus of nutritional research and medical concern. In the meantime, beware of writers and diet gurus who use it to justify their recommendations to eliminate or drastically reduce consumption of carbohydrate foods. Eating a lot of high-GI carbohydrates will worsen your situation if you are insulin resistant; it will not make you insulin resistant. (There is even a bit of experimental evidence suggesting that very high carbohydrate diets actually increase the effectiveness of insulin slightly.)

You might well ask, If so much of the theory behind the low-carbohydrate diets is wrong, why do people lose weight on them, and do the diets represent a healthy way to eat?

Let me recount two stories of dieters, both friends, who talked to me recently about experiences in eliminating most carbohydrates from their diets. The first, a woman in her early fifties, is very active with generally healthy habits. Though far from obese, she has struggled for years to lose ten to fifteen pounds that she considers excessive, employing a variety of unsuccessful reducing diets and exercise programs. She told me she had been on a low-carbohydrate diet for three weeks and had lost six pounds—"the first time I've been able to lose any weight at all, and I'm eating bacon, and salad dressings, and all the cheese I want, everything I haven't let myself have in years. How can this be?" she asked. She is strictly avoiding bread, pasta, other starches, and sugar. "Sugar is a big one for me," she said, "because I really love sweets, but now I'm finding that with no sugar in my diet, fruit is overwhelmingly sensual; a slice of watermelon is voluptuous."

My other friend, a businessman also in his fifties, who is genuinely overweight, addicted to exercise in gyms, and a longtime devotee of low-fat "spa" cuisine, recently went on the Atkins diet. I went with him to a Sunday buffet brunch at a resort in California, where he had just finished a three-hour workout on aerobics machines and weights. He returned from the buffet with a plate (the first of several) loaded to overflowing with ham, bacon, sausages, steak, cheese, and scrambled eggs, which he devoured with gusto and confidence that his weight would soon be dropping. "This is great," he told me between plates. He put artificial sweetener in his coffee and was careful not to let a single morsel of carbohydrate pass his lips.

I told the first friend to keep me informed of her progress. At last notice, she was still on a low-carbohydrate diet, still losing weight (she dropped one dress size), and still missing sweets. I will be interested to see how long she can stay on this regimen and what will happen when she alters it. My second friend was not ready to hear any advice about his food choices, such as the possibility that his caloric intake had gone way up on his new regime of eating only fat and protein, but when I saw him again a month later, he was "off Atkins," no slimmer, and bouncing back and forth between low-fat and low-carbohydrate meal plans. He struck me as totally confused about the right way to eat.

I devote a whole chapter to the subject of losing weight later in this book, but here is my take on this kind of dieting: There is no question that people can lose weight by shunning carbohydrates. The reasons for this weight loss are interesting and subtle. If you stop eating carbohydrates, your body will quickly use its stores of glycogen in the liver to maintain blood glucose for the brain and in the muscles to power activity. Glycogen is hydrophilic, meaning it loves water and binds water to itself when it is stored in tissues. In fact, it binds two to three times its own weight of water, meaning that when glycogen stores are full, several pounds of water are stored along with it. This water is released and excreted in urine as glycogen stores are depleted. This happens fast, and dieters are delighted to see the results they want in spite of eating foods they have always been told are fattening. It is important to keep in mind, though, that the intial loss of weight on a low- or no-carbohydrate diet—usually five or six pounds—is water that will be gained back as soon as you resume eating starch or sugar.

Further weight loss on these diets involves different mechanisms. One possibility is that the metabolic processing of fat and, especially, protein as energy sources is less efficient than that of carbohydrate, meaning the body has to expend more calories to get the calories from fat and protein than from carbohydrate. But I think a likelier explanation is reduced caloric intake as a result of the monotony of the diet and the satiating effect of high-fat meals.

People will lose weight on any monotonous diet, because the food becomes boring, and incentive to eat diminishes. I am quite sure that I could promote an all-cheesecake diet that would work for some: eat all the cheesecake you can at every meal but only cheesecake. Within a short time the idea of sitting down to another helping of cheesecake would become so unappealing that you would eat very little. Your intake of calories would drop and so would weight. In my experience, high-fat foods become boring more quickly than high-carbohydrate foods, so cheesecake would be a good choice for this regime, especially because it is a classic forbidden food on standard reducing diets.

I can't prove that this boredom with food is the main reason people continue to lose weight on the Atkins diet and similar regimes once they pass through the water-loss phase, but I can recount a personal experience that was very convincing to me. In the spring of 1961, I was finishing my first year of college in Cambridge, Massachusetts, during my pre-health-conscious days, when I did not exercise, ate everything and anything, and was overweight. One morning, shortly before the start of final exams, as I was walking down Massachusetts Avenue toward Harvard Square, I saw that the entire window of a bookstore was filled with a display of a new book and posters about it: *Calories Don't Count* by Herman Taller, M.D. I, who believed that calories did count and that the only way to lose weight was to take in fewer of them, was hooked. I entered the store, browsed the book, bought it, and headed back to my room. I read it in one sitting.

Taller was an early preacher of the no-carbohydrate approach to weight loss. No one talked about insulin resistance or glycemic index back then, but Taller had a gimmick. He wrote that some fats were bad and some were good, a fact I agree with as I will explain in the next chapter, but the particular fat he chose to promote was one few people had heard of in 1961—safflower oil. Safflower oil, from the seed of a plant in the daisy family native to India, is a polyunsaturated oil; in fact, it has the highest content of polyunsaturated fatty acids of all the edible oils. In 1961, the medical community was in agreement that saturated fats were bad and was beginning to promote the use of polyunsaturated oils and margarines made from them. Taller put his own spin on this. He wrote that safflower oil had a special, almost magical ability to stimulate the body to burn stored fat, and the more of it you could consume, the faster your body would eliminate excess fat, calories be damned.

The meal plan recommended in his book was a no-carbohydrate, high-protein diet emphasizing safflower oil. You were supposed to cook everything in it, pour it on salads, take capsules of it, and even—if you could stand it—drink jiggers of it with meals. Bookstores conveniently offered bottles of safflower oil and safflower oil capsules along with the book, an early example of a kind of promotional marketing of books and products that has since become commonplace. Of course, I went back to the bookstore for my supplies of magic oil, since I had determined to try the diet. Not only did it sound easy, the idea of eating fat with abandon was very seductive after having spent so much time trying to resist the temptations of high-fat foods.

Putting the theories contained in *Calories Don't Count* into practice did not turn out to be so easy, in part because of the limitations of life in an ancient college dormitory. I had no cooking facilities, only a hot plate, and the grocery stores in the vicinity were of the minimalist sort. Unable to prepare or cook anything elaborate, I settled on the following plan. For breakfast, I ate a can of tuna fish with safflower oil dressing, and for both lunch and dinner, I had sliced knockwurst that I fried in ample safflower oil on my hot plate, accompanied by a green salad (mostly iceberg lettuce, as that was all I could get) tossed with more safflower oil and vinegar. Dutifully, I drank a jigger of safflower oil with lunch and dinner. If you have never tried to drink vegetable oil by the jigger, you can't imagine how challenging it is.

After three days on this regimen, I noticed a number of changes. First, I alienated my roommates, who complained of the smell of fried knockwurst and the pall of greasy smoke that became permanent features of our suite of rooms. Second, my appetite declined rapidly. In fact, by the third day, the thought of sitting down to another of my lunches or dinners was disgusting, and I actually felt a bit of nausea on raising the jigger of oil to my lips. Third, my hands were so oily that I had to be careful about getting grease stains on whatever I touched. Fourth, however, my weight dropped by several pounds, which was tremendously encouraging and reinforced my intention to persevere. Clearly, Dr. Taller was onto something not known to conventional medical science.

By this time I was in the midst of exams, staying up late into the night to cram, sleeping irregularly, and not being able to socialize, because most social events were organized around eating and drinking foods and beverages I could not have. I lived this way for one week, at the end of which I had lost eleven pounds. I was also in a terrible mood, listless, grouchy, and ready to choke if I had to drink another jigger of safflower oil. My roommates gave me constant abuse. When I finished my last final exam late on a Friday afternoon and was turning in my blue book, I was horrified to see that its cover and inside pages were translucent with grease from my fingers. "Enough of this," I said to myself. I swept up my roommates to go into Boston to a favorite delicatessen restaurant, where I ate everything and anything, finishing with an ice-cream sundae. I came home to fall into a stuporous sleep. When I got up the next morning, I discovered that I had regained all eleven pounds overnight!

In my experience most people use the Atkins diet for short-term weight loss—to get into a new swimsuit, for example, or to counteract the effects of holiday gluttony. For this purpose and short duration, I suppose it is harmless, except insofar as it contributes to cyclic weight loss and gain ("yo-yo dieting") that ultimately contributes to worse and more stubborn obesity. But as a long-term strategy, either for weight control or fitness, I do not consider it healthy to keep carbohydrates out of the diet or reduce them to minimal levels.

Putting aside the detrimental effects of replacing carbohydrate with excessive fat and protein, which I will discuss in the following chapters, depriving the body of its highest-quality fuel reduces the efficiency of digestion and metabolism, makes it harder to replenish glycogen stores, and may encourage the breakdown of muscle tissue. Moreover, it removes from the diet foods that establish cultural identity, reinforce social connection, and provide satisfaction as well as sustenance. Think about how many enjoyable, common comfort foods are carbohydrates: toast, baked potatoes, and rice pudding, for example.

But, while I reject the theories and nutritional philosophies of Atkins, Montignac, Sears, and their adherents, I am very concerned about how much and what kinds of carbohydrate belong in the optimum diet and how current patterns of carbohydrate consumption influence health.

Most dietitians recommend that at least 50 and at most 60 percent of calories come from carbohydrates, but except for telling us to eat more complex carbohydrates and fewer simple ones, they have little else to say. I agree with the general percentages, which translate out to about 125 to 150 grams of carbohydrate a day for every 1,000 calories in your diet. A moderately active woman aged eighteen to fifty-four would eat about 1,800 calories a day, of which 900 to 1,080 should come from carbohydrate, that is, 225 to 270 grams of carbohydrate a day. Her male counterpart, needing about 2,300 calories a day, should get 1,150 to 1,380 carbohydrate calories or 288 to 345 grams of carbohydrate a day.

I also want to make these strong recommendations:

- The majority of carbohydrate calories should come from less refined, less processed foods with low-glycemic-index ratings. Processed foods tend to be unhealthy in several ways: They are low in fiber and other protective micronutrients, and often high in sodium and the wrong kinds of fat, so eating less of them is a good idea in general as well as for any specific effect on carbohydrate metabolism.

- It is desirable to eat some low-GI carbohydrate with most meals, such as whole grains, beans, vegetables, and low-GI fruits (generally temperate fruits like berries, apples, and cherries as opposed to tropical ones like mangoes, papayas, and pineapples).

- If you eat high-GI foods, eat them in moderate quantities and balance them by adding some low-GI foods at the same meal.
- Reduce the impact of high-GI foods by eating them as part of mixed meals, including fiber and acid (lemon juice and vinegar).
- Minimize consumptions of foods and beverages sweetened with high-fructose corn syrup. These tend to be low-quality foods, and you are better off using less of them. Also, do not use pure, granulated fructose as a substitute for table sugar.
- Make an effort to replace white and whole-wheat bread with dense, chewy, grainy breads whenever possible.
- Learn to like firmer-cooked (*al dente*) pasta rather than longer-cooked.
- Eat more small, waxy, new potatoes and fewer large, floury potatoes.
- Eat more basmati and converted rice and less regular or sticky rice.
- Eat more beans. They are high-quality foods providing low-GI carbohydrate along with other nutrients.

These recommendations apply to all of us, but are especially important if you have symptoms of insulin resistance, adult-onset diabetes, obesity, cardiovascular disease, elevated blood fats (serum lipids or triglycerides), or have a family history of these problems.

Finally, although low-carbohydrate diets may work for short-term weight loss, they are not the healthiest strategy for losing weight, and I do not recommend them as an everyday way to eat. That does not mean that I endorse low-fat diets, either. Those regimens present different problems, which I will explain in the next section. But first I want to give you a bit more information about fats in general.

III

FAT REVISITED:
THE BEST PART OF FOOD OR THE WORST?

We have such bad associations to the word *fat* these days that it is difficult even to think of positive usages. But a few linger on, such as *fat city* as a term for a good place to be. I once heard a music critic aptly describe the beautiful melody of the third movement of

Brahms's Double Concerto as "fat and sunny." Most people in the Western world regard body fat as something to get rid of, and the cultures who hold a different view, like Hawaiians, are fast disappearing. Gypsies also equate ample body fat with prosperity and happiness; they are decidedly out of the cultural mainstream in the countries they inhabit.

Because it is the most calorie-dense of the macronutrients, fat has a very positive potential, especially for people facing scarcity. Think again of our Paleolithic ancestors, who certainly knew both feast and famine. When they killed and cooked large animals, the fat of the meat would have comprised the choicest cuts, providing them with caloric insurance against lean times ahead. I once visited a group of Inuit in the Canadian Arctic at the northern end of Baffin Island and watched them hunt seals and small whales and eat fresh blubber from the kills with the greatest delight. They simply cut it out of the carcasses and passed out portions to everyone present. The Inuit's love of fat, even raw, unadorned fat from marine mammals, is unique and probably necessary for their survival in a cold, harsh land. It is also a graphic example of the preference for fat we have inherited from our hunter-gatherer ancestors.

The fact is that fat tastes good to us. It accounts for much of the flavor of food and also contributes to an all-important quality of "mouth feel" that food technologists pay great attention to. Chocolate is appealing to so many of us in part because of the sensuous mouth feel of cocoa butter. Indian cooks begin the preparation of most dishes by frying whole, dried spices in clarified butter (ghee) to release their flavors. Many of the flavor components of spices and other foods are fat-soluble, and fat is the vehicle that conveys them to our taste buds. Most people find the combination of positive mouth feel and concentration of flavor irresistible. When we describe food we like as "rich," we are usually responding to the pleasure provided by its content of fat. Compare the experience of eating a handful of your favorite potato or corn chips to one of their fat-free counterparts.

I believe we respond positively to this experience as a result of natural selection. Just as preference for sweetness guided early humans to sources of instant energy that increased chances of survival, so did preference for fat lead them to sources of concentrated calories that would have done the same. Most of us have inherited a "fat tooth" as well as a sweet tooth and for equally good evolutionary reasons. The bottom line is that we like fat, and advice to eat less of it runs up against the simple fact that fat accounts for much of the pleasure we experience from food. It is not impossible, but certainly difficult, to make fat-free and low-fat versions of favorite dishes taste as good as the originals. People on low-fat diets often find it hard to enjoy the social experience of dining. And the particular fat we use significantly contributes to the role of food in defining cultural identity—ghee for Indians, olive oil for peoples of the Mediterranean region, butter for northern and western Europeans.

Can something we like so much be so bad for us? Is fat really the chief culprit in the modern diet, the cause of, or main contributor to, obesity, heart disease, and cancer? In my view, as is the case with carbohydrate, fat per se is not the problem. The problem is the kinds of fat that have become dominant in our diets. In order to explain why I hold that opinion and to tell you how much of what kind of fat the optimum diet should contain, I must first give you some more background information about lipids (fats, oils, fatty acids, and compounds derived from them)—how they exist in our bodies, how they move about, and what specialized functions they perform.

Very little fat in the body exists as free fatty acids. Most fatty acids are hooked together, three at a time, onto a carrier molecule, glycerol. Glycerol is a simple compound of carbon, hydrogen, and oxygen easily derived from the metabolic breakdown of glucose. Its three carbon atoms serve as a backbone to which fatty acid chains can be linked; these combinations are called triglycerides.* The fat stored in our fat cells is in the form of triglycerides, as is most of the fat moving through the bloodstream. Triglycerides also comprise the main type of fat in food, accounting for 95 percent of the fat we eat.

The outside carbons of a glycerol molecule prefer to hold saturated fatty acids (SFAs), while the middle carbon prefers an unsaturated fatty acid (MUFA or PUFA), but this varies from food to food. Artificially hydrogenated fats (like vegetable shortening), which I will have a lot more to say about, have SFAs on all positions, while some seed oils have PUFAs in all positions. Given the varying lengths and degrees of saturation of different fatty-acid molecules and the three positions available for attachment, there are a great many possible

---

*Biochemists object to this term because it is inaccurate chemically. They want us to talk about *triacylglycerols*, or *TAGs*. But in medical usage *triglycerides* is universal, and that is the term I will use.

permutations. All fats and oils are mostly mixtures of different triglycerides. When we eat them, the body frees the fatty acids from their glycerol carriers and rearranges them into new triglycerides for its own uses. Stored triglycerides in the body's fatty (adipose) tissue are primarily reserves of calories; to get to those calories, the body again separates the fatty acids (primarily SFAs and MUFAs) from glycerol and sends them to sites of cellular oxidation, where they are burned for energy. Stored triglycerides are also reserves of essential fatty acids (EFAs), the special PUFAs needed for critically important structural and regulatory roles in the body.

SATURATED FATS AND OILS (SFAS)	MONOUNSATURATED OILS (MUFAS)	POLYUNSATURATED OILS (PUFAS)
Animal fat	Avocado oil	Corn oil
Butter fat	Canola oil	Cottonseed oil
Coconut oil	Olive oil	Fish oil
Palm kernel oil	Peanut oil	Flaxseed oil
Palm oil		Grapeseed oil
		Safflower oil
		Sesame oil
		Soybean oil
		Sunflower oil
		Walnut oil

One of the most common medical diagnostic tests ordered today is the serum lipid profile to measure levels of fat and cholesterol in the blood. It includes a determination of serum triglycerides. High levels result from overeating, especially from eating too much refined carbohydrate with high glycemic index. High serum triglycerides are associated with increased risk of heart disease (especially in women), because they often signal abnormal lipid metabolism and arterial damage.

Most of the serum lipid profile concerns cholesterol, a hard, waxy substance that occurs in many animal foods (especially meat, whole milk, and egg yolks) and is also made by the liver. Cholesterol performs vital functions in the body. It serves as the starting material for the synthesis of important hormones—sex hormones like estrogen and testosterone, and adrenal hormones such as cortisone that regulate metabolism. The body derives vitamin D, necessary for utilization of calcium, and makes bile acids from cholesterol. Bile acids aid the digestion of dietary fats by breaking them down into smaller particles, and the body can rid itself of excess cholesterol by adding it to bile that is secreted into the small intestine during digestion. Cholesterol is also a component of the secretions of oil glands that protect the skin from dehydration and other sorts of environmental irritation.

Finally, cholesterol is vitally important as a modifier of the structure of cell membranes. Recall that cell membranes are mostly composed of lipids. The unsaturated essential fatty acids make membranes more flexible, while more saturated fatty acids make them stiffer. Day-to-day variations in the intake of fatty acids create a problem in maintaining flexibility of cell membranes within the narrow limits necessary for optimum health. The body uses cholesterol to compensate for these variations, adding more to stiffen membranes that are too fluid and removing some to soften ones that are too stiff.

If cholesterol is important to the body in so many ways, why does it have such a bad reputation? The reason is that it is also the main component of arterial plaque, the hallmark of atherosclerosis, responsible for the stiffening and narrowing of arteries that lead to heart attacks, strokes, and other circulatory calamities. There is no question that atherosclerosis is pathological, that a disorder of cholesterol production and transport is central to it, and that it is a disease of modern, urbanized society greatly influenced by diet. But many questions remain, among them, just what dietary excesses or deficiencies cause cholesterol production and transport to go awry?

I noted earlier that the liver makes cholesterol as a component of bile. The adrenal glands and sex glands make it to produce their hormones, and virtually all cells manufacture small amounts for their own membrane requirements. In order to make cholesterol the body starts with the two-carbon fragments—acetate fragments—produced by fatty acid oxidation, the breakdown and burning of fats as fuel. Since SFAs are the preferred fuel fats, SFAs are the main source of acetate fragments, but the burning of carbohydrates also produces them as intermediate products of metabolism before full transformation to carbon dioxide and water.

Diets high in saturated fat and high-glycemic-index carbohydrates lead to increased production of acetate fragments in the body, and an excess of acetate fragments, in most people, drives production of cholesterol. (I say "most people" because cholesterol production, like other aspects of metabolism, is also influenced by genetics. Some lucky people have inherited so-called Methuselah genes that keep them from producing excess cholesterol and developing atherosclerosis no matter how much saturated fat and refined carbohydrate they eat.) We also get cholesterol from our food, in lesser or greater quantity, depending on the percentage of animal foods we eat, but cholesterol that we eat has a relatively slight influence on the serum lipid profile compared to the effect of saturated fat and refined sugars and starches. For years, egg producers have complained that eggs have gotten a bad rap in all the fuss about cholesterol, and they are right. Egg yolks contain cholesterol, but their inclusion in the diet makes an insignificant contribution to serum cholesterol; besides, they can be an important source of the scarce essential fatty acids.

Increased cholesterol production is only one part of the story of atherosclerosis. Equally important is the way this substance moves around the body. Triglycerides and cholesterol move through the blood together in protein-coated droplets called lipoproteins of varying size and function. Lipoproteins are transport vehicles made by the liver for conveying lipids to and from cells. When tiny fat droplets from the intestinal digestion of dietary fat enter the bloodstream after a meal, they are taken up by one class of lipoproteins called high-density lipoproteins or HDL. HDL conveys triglycerides and cholesterol to the liver. The liver can metabolize them further, send them out to other parts of the body, or, in the case of cholesterol, eliminate it in bile. If it sends them out, it does so in another class of transport vehicles called LDL, or low-density lipoproteins.

You may have heard the terms *good cholesterol* and *bad cholesterol* applied to HDL and LDL. In fact, HDL and LDL are simply carriers or transport vehicles, not just for cholesterol but also for triglycerides, and both are needed to move these substances around the body. All cells have specialized receptors for LDL on their membranes, docking sites where these transport vehicles can land to unload their cargo. In this way cells get the fats and cholesterol they need for their functions. When those needs are met, the docks close, and excess fats and cholesterol continue to circulate as LDL in the blood until their contents are taken to fat cells for storage or transferred to HDL for return to the liver.

High levels of LDL in the blood, low levels of HDL, and a low HDL to LDL ratio are all correlated with atherosclerosis and increased risk of heart attack. Genetic inheritance determines a great deal of our individual lipoprotein profile, some unlucky persons having familial hyperlipidemias (high blood fats) that are not much influenced by diet, while the few lucky ones with Methusaleh genes are able to clear fats and cholesterol from the blood efficiently no matter what they eat.

In most of us, eating a lot of the wrong fats and carbohydrates will elevate serum triglycerides and cholesterol, increase LDL transport of fats and cholesterol to tissues, and overwhelm the capacity of HDL to bring the excess back to the liver. In the form of LDL, cholesterol can damage the walls of arteries, but whether it does so or not depends on other factors. I will mention a few of them as a way of emphasizing that the whole story of atherosclerosis remains to be told.

One possible factor is that some kind of damage to the walls of arteries must occur first in order for cholesterol to deposit there. More and more medical experts are coming to believe that the underlying problem is inflammation, caused by imbalances in the hormones that mediate the inflammatory response or even by a bacterial infection.* Some even suggest that the presence of cholesterol in arterial plaque represents a flawed healing response, an attempt by the body to repair defects in vessel walls. Another possibility is that some forms of cholesterol are directly damaging to arteries. Roving white blood cells (macrophages) gobble up oxidized cholesterol and thereby transform themselves into "foam cells" that attach to artery walls and may initiate a process of inflammation and degeneration. The susceptibility of cholesterol to oxidation is influenced by the nature of the fats that travel with it in LDL. For example, if your principal dietary fat is olive oil, your LDL will contain triglycerides rich in oleic acid, the MUFA in olive oil. Traveling in that company, cholesterol is relatively protected from oxidation. So although the correlation between high serum LDL and heart disease risk is clear, as are the benefits of lowering serum LDL by drugs or lifestyle mea-

---

*The organism *Chlamydia pneumoniae*, found in high frequency in atherosclerotic plaque, is now suspected as a cause of the problem. If atherosclerosis and coronary artery disease turn out to be infectious in origin, that will be a major revolution in medical thinking. It will also create possibilities for preventing and treating these problems with specific antimicrobial agents.

sures, the cause-and-effect sequence between high LDL cholesterol and atherosclerosis is not. In some circumstances, and in some individuals, high levels of so-called bad cholesterol may not cause damage.

Given all this uncertainty, it is more than a little risky to blame diet alone for the epidemic of heart attacks in developed countries in this century, but it is important to look at a possible connection if we are trying to decide how much and what kind of fat we should eat. At the beginning of the century, death from heart attack was an uncommon event. It became all too common in the 1940s, 1950s, and 1960s, felling many middle-aged men and post-menopausal women. The same pattern occurred in other industrialized countries but generally was not seen in the Third World. Since the late 1960s the epidemic of heart attacks has waned, for reasons as mysterious as those accounting for its rise.

One possibility is that increased use of antibiotics has treated many unrecognized bacterial infections in human arteries. Another theory is that increased use of aspirin has given many people protection against the blood clots that are the immediate cause of coronary artery obstructions. (Blood tends to clot on roughened surfaces of plaque, especially if plaque ruptures.) Still other possibilities are the emergence of effective drug treatments for hypertension, a known risk factor for cardiovascular disease, and the decline in smoking among men. But many epidemiologists continue to look to dietary explanations for both the rise and fall of coronary heart disease in the twentieth century.

We can see that as peoples of other countries begin to eat the way we do, their rates of coronary heart disease go up. That is a clear pattern in contemporary Japan and China, for example. So there must be something about the Western diet that promotes arterial damage.

It is tempting to think that the problem is saturated fat, especially in meat, milk, cream, ice cream, butter, and cheese, all foods absent from the traditional diets of China, Japan, and other Asian countries where heart attacks were once rare to the point of being medical curiosities. Breakfast in Japan used to include miso soup, steamed rice, a piece of broiled fish (often salmon), pickled and cooked vegetables, dried seaweed, and green tea. Today it is likely to be scrambled eggs and bacon, toasted white bread with butter, pastry, and coffee with cream and sugar—quite a change. As I mentioned earlier, we know also that during the German occupation of Holland, Denmark, and Norway in World War II, deaths from heart attack plummeted as animal foods became scarce. They rose to prewar levels after the war when those foods again became available.

But there must be more to the story, because Americans were eating a lot of saturated fat throughout the nineteenth century and the early years of the twentieth century and not having heart attacks. They were also eating plenty of refined flour and sugar. What changed? Why didn't traditional Inuit suffer from coronary heart disease when they were eating so much animal fat?

Some experts, and all of the antifat camp, tell us that the total amount of fat we eat is the main determinant of health and longevity: The higher the percentage of fat calories in the diet, the shorter the life span and greater the risks of disease in general, not just heart disease. But both research and epidemiological surveys fail to support this position. Science has established a direct correlation between saturated fat intake and LDL cholesterol in the blood. Most people who eat more saturated fat will have more LDL cholesterol and, unless they are protected by other factors (genetics, exercise, and aspirin among them) will have higher risks of cardiovascular disease. Science has established no such correlation for total fat intake and disease risks.

If you look for those correlations in Europe today, you are in for some surprises, especially if you subscribe to the Ornish/Pritikin philosophy or the spa mentality that rules in many health-care institutions. Scotland, with the highest intake of both total fat and saturated fat, has staggering rates of cardiovascular disease, just what you would expect. (The latest contribution of Scotland to world cuisine is deep-fried Mars bars: candy bars dipped in batter, fried, and served as dessert in the fish-and-chips shops.) But in parts of Italy and Spain, in Greece, and on the island of Crete, people are eating comparable amounts of total fat and not dying of heart attacks (or getting other degenerative diseases or cancer) at higher than expected rates. Cretans eat 40 percent of their calories as fat, which rivals Americans and Scots, and are much healthier. The fats they eat are quite different, however.

These observations draw attention to the possibility that the kinds of fat in the diet may be more important than total fat. Saturated fats can be unhealthy, but that may be true of other fats as well. And some fats might actually promote health. What I intend to do is look at distinctions between good and bad fats and changes in proportions of them in people's diets over the past century. As I do so, be aware that merely talking about good fats and bad fats raises the hackles of Ornish/Pritikin followers, who believe that fat always equates with bad.

In the 1950s, when the scientific consensus was that saturated fat raises cholesterol levels and heart attack risks, doctors and dietitians began warning people away from beef, butter, cream, and cheese, and urging them to use polyunsaturated vegetable oils in the belief that these were heart healthy. This was the era of the skyrocketing popularity of margarine made from corn oil and booming sales of vegetable oils from a variety of sources including cottonseeds and peanuts. Common sense seemed to support these recommendations in that saturated fats are solid or semisolid at body temperature whereas polyunsaturated oils are liquid. One would expect solid fats to leave sludgy residues and liquid oils to move freely in blood vessels. Unfortunately, common sense did not alert us to the dangers in the vegetable oils that have become so prevalent in our diets. To discuss those dangers I must give you a bit more background on the chemistry of fats and oils.

Recall that fatty acids are straight chains of carbon atoms with hydrogen atoms attached. One end of a fatty acid molecule, usually thought of as the beginning, because synthesis begins there, is a methyl group—a carbon atom with three attached hydrogens. The other end is a carboxyl group, the oxygen-containing portion of the molecule that gives it a weakly acid nature. By convention, the carbon atoms of a fatty acid molecule are numbered, beginning from the methyl end. SFAs are identified very simply by specifying the number of carbons in the chain; since no double bonds are present, the structure of the molecule is known. Thus stearic acid, found in the fat of many animals, is designated in chemical shorthand as C18:0, meaning a fatty acid chain eighteen carbons long with zero double bonds, hence an SFA.

In chemical notation, the presence of a double bond is indicated by the Greek letter ω (omega), and its position in the chain by the number of the first carbon atom that participates in it. Oleic acid, the main fatty acid in olive oil, is the same length as stearic acid but contains one double bond between carbons 9 and 10; therefore, it is designated $C18:1\omega9$, a MUFA (*mono*unsaturated fatty acid—one double bond) belonging to the omega-9 series, a small family of fatty acids with the first double bond in the 9–10 position. Linoleic acid, one of the essential fatty acids, is another $C18$ chain, but a PUFA (*poly*unsaturated fatty acid—more than one double bond) with two double bonds, one in the 6–7 position, the other in the 9–10 position. It is $C18:2\omega6$ in the omega-6 series, an important family, which I will have much to say about. (For PUFAs, you need only specify the position of the first double bond, for reasons I need not explain here.) The other essential fatty acid, linolenic acid, is $C18:3\omega3$. This shorthand name tells you that linolenic acid is an eighteen-carbon PUFA, containing three double bonds, the first between carbons 3 and 4. Linolenic acid is therefore an omega-3 fatty acid. I have already told you about the importance of that family.

When plants and animals synthesize fatty acids from glucose, they first make SFAs, adding two-carbon units end to end until the desired chain length is reached and terminated with a carboxyl group. They can then use enzymes at particular positions of the chain to create MUFAs and PUFAs. But there is an important difference between these biological kingdoms with respect to fatty acid synthesis: While plants can insert double bonds near the beginnings of fatty acid chains (in the omega-3 and omega-6 positions, for example), animals cannot. Animals can put double bonds farther down the line but not up front; they lack the enzymes to do so. Yet they need both omega-3 and omega-6 fatty acids for important functions and will become sick and even die without them. That is why linolenic and linoleic acids are essential: You must have them in your diet and have them regularly to live and be healthy.

Wait a minute, you might say, I've told you that fish like salmon and sardines are important sources of omega-3 fatty acids and that egg yolks can provide EFAs. Aren't fish and chickens members of the animal kingdom? Of course they are, and they cannot manufacture omega-3 fatty acids any more than we can. But they can eat them and store them. Salmon and sardines get them by eating algae and other simple forms of plant life that make omega-3s, then store them in their body fat. Chickens in the wild can find plant sources of omega-3s to put in the yolks of their eggs.

When salmon and chickens are farmed, the omega-3 content of foods derived from them is determined by what they get to eat.

Unless salmon farmers make an effort to provide dietary sources of omega-3s, the flesh of farmed salmon will be much inferior to that of wild salmon as a source of essential fatty acids. Chickens confined to cages eating standard feed will not produce eggs that have anywhere near the omega-3 content of eggs of free-range chickens that scratch and peck the ground for food. Recently, a new egg has appeared on the American market, one high in omega-3 fatty acids. Egg farmers get this result by fortifying chicken feed with a meal made from algae. In the same way, animals that eat plant sources of essential fatty acids (EFAs), either directly or indirectly (fish, eggs), will have high levels of EFAs in their body fat. Vegetarians tend to have significantly higher levels of stored EFAs than meat eaters, for example.

Animals deprived of linoleic acid (LA) in experiments develop a syndrome marked by skin inflammation, hair loss, liver and kidney degeneration, decreased healing response, and increased susceptibility to infection, cardiovascular problems, behavioral disturbances, arthritis, growth retardation, and, eventually, death. All symptoms reverse if LA is restored to the diet. Removal of linolenic acid (LNA) results in a different deficiency syndrome that includes growth retardation, weakness, lack of coordination, behavioral changes, and impairment of learning ability. LA has been studied far more than LNA, but I believe it is fair to say that we still do not fully understand the functions of either of these essential fatty acids in maintaining life and health. What we do know is that both are vital to the production of energy from food and movement of energy to all systems of the body, that they regulate transport of oxygen, that they are critical to the integrity and function of membranes, and that they are the starting materials for the synthesis of prostaglandins, hormones that govern many basic life processes, including the healing response.

There is growing medical awareness that essential fatty acid deficiency may be widespread and very detrimental to both physical and mental well-being. We do not see in humans the full-blown deficiency syndromes that occur in experimental animals given no dietary EFAs, but human diseases that may be caused or aggravated by relative EFA deficiency are very common and include atherosclerosis and coronary heart disease. One indirect piece of evidence that must be very upsetting to the antifat camp is a recent finding of the ongoing Harvard Nurses' Health Study, established in 1976 to examine the relationship between diet and disease. Women in the study who regularly ate mayonnaise and oil-based salad dressings had greatly reduced risks of fatal coronary heart disease compared to women who ate those foods rarely. The researchers argued that mayonnaise and salad dressings can be sources of LNA, the heart-protective EFA.

Instead of talking about EFA deficiency, nutritionists should really focus on omega-3 deficiency, because LA, the omega-6 fatty acid, is plentiful, both in nature and in our diets. Not only is it in many seeds and nuts, it is in the oils expressed from them, including all of the polyunsaturated vegetable oils on the market, and it accumulates in the fat of some animals, especially pigs. On the other hand LNA, the parent omega-3 EFA, occurs in only a few seeds and nuts (flax, hemp, pumpkin, and walnuts) and fewer oils (canola and soy, which may account for the benefits of salad dressings in the Harvard Nurses' Study report). Thus many plants produce seeds full of omega-6 EFAs, but very few have omega-3s there. Instead, omega-3 EFAs abound in microscopic forms of plant life, like algae; in higher plants they tend to occur in leaves, although usually in low concentrations. (See the chart on page 85.)

One unusual plant with a respectable content of omega-3 EFAs in its leaves is purslane (*Portulaca oleracea*), a little plant with succulent (fleshy) leaves that many gardeners know as an invasive pest. Mediterranean peoples value purslane, adding its leaves to soups. Mexicans, who call it *verdolagas,* sauté it with onions or chop it into fresh salsa with tomatoes, onions, and chilies. It is easy to grow, and improved forms are available from specialty seed suppliers.

Dark leafy greens also supply omega-3 EFAs, again not in high concentration, but this may be one reason that cooked greens are a healthy addition to the diet. (They also supply folic acid, a key vitamin in the B-complex group, along with other micronutrients.) Wild grasses are another source of these necessary fats, and while we do not eat grass, we do consume the flesh of grazing animals that eat it in quantity. That brings us to an interesting consideration about how the modern diet has changed for the worse.

Our Paleolithic ancestors ate a lot of foods of animal origin, including fish, fowl, and large mammals. The fat of these animals was full of EFAs, especially omega-3 EFAs from the grasses and other plants in their diets. Scientists interested in the virtues of the Paleolithic diet estimate that it provided the two classes of EFAs—the

OMEGA-3 SOURCES	OMEGA-6 SOURCES
Fish oil	Corn oil
Flaxseed oil	Cottonseed oil
Flax seeds	Grapeseed oil
Hemp seeds	Meat
Herring	Peanut oil
Mackerel	Poultry
Purslane	Safflower oil
Salmon	Sesame oil
Sardines	Soybean oil
Soybean oil*	Sunflower oil
Soybeans	
Walnut oil	
Walnuts	

*Note: Soybean oil is higher in omega-6 fatty acids than most omega-3 oils, so it belongs in both categories.

omega-6 and the omega-3—in about equal proportions. Flesh foods in the modern diet are very different because so many animals raised for food today, including chickens, pigs, cows, and sheep, no longer graze in the wild. Instead, most are fattened with grains such as corn that provide LA (omega-6) but not LNA (omega-3). Moreover, people take in a lot of their fat in the form of vegetable oils and products like margarine made from them; most of these, again, provide omega-6 fatty acids, but not omega-3s. Estimates of the ratio of omega-6 to omega-3 fatty acids in the modern diet are between twenty-to-one and forty-to-one, a huge change from what our distant ancestors ate. This may well have consequences for human health and longevity.

I have said that the body must have both of these EFAs on a regular basis. Once it has a fatty acid with a double bond in the 6–7 position, an omega-6, it can make other needed fatty acids in that series by changing the length of the chain or adding other double bonds down the line. It can do the same with a fatty acid containing a double bond in the 3–4 position, an omega-3; for instance, EPA (eicosapentaenoic acid), one of the key components of salmon and sardine oil that has a protective effect on the heart, can be made from LNA. However, the body cannot make it if it has no starting material with a double bond in the 3–4 position. And even if it has the right starting material, it cannot make EPA if there are too many omega-6 fatty acids in the diet.

The problem is that as the ratio of omega-6s to omega-3s increases, the efficiency of those omega-3s that are available declines, because both types of fatty acids compete for the same limited supply of enzymes. Therefore, the ratio of omega-6s to omega-3s in the diet may strongly influence the behavior of essential fatty acids in the body. For one key function—the synthesis of prostaglandin hormones—that ratio appears to be critically important.

It is beyond the scope of this book to detail the synthesis and effects of prostaglandins. Suffice it to say that they govern all cell growth and differentiation, blood clotting, and key aspects of immune function. Unlike insulin and other endocrine hormones, prostaglandins are not made in particular glands like the pancreas, where they are stored until needed. Instead, all cells in the body (except red blood cells) synthesize them from EFAs on demand for immediate release.

A century ago the Bayer pharmaceutical company in Germany invented aspirin, a semisynthetic derivative of salicylic acid, found naturally in willow bark. (Native Americans used to brew white willow bark into a tea for treatment of fever and arthritis.) The new drug quickly established itself as an effective remedy for fever, pain, and inflammation, but for most of the past century its mechanism of action was unknown. Aspirin has so many apparently unrelated effects on the body that no one could make sense of how it worked—until the discovery of prostaglandins. Aspirin modulates these hormones, and its myriad actions are mediated by them.

Much more recently, doctors discovered that aspirin thins the blood and began recommending that people take it every day to lower their risk of heart attack. (I take two baby aspirins a day—162 milligrams, equal to half of a regular tablet.) Most doctors assume this prescription works by reducing the clotting tendency of the blood so that even if coronary arteries are narrowed and roughened by atherosclerosis, blood clots are less likely to form in them. But some experts now suggest that the anti-inflammatory action of aspirin is the real explanation, assuming that atherosclerosis is fundamentally an inflammatory disorder of arteries. Meanwhile, daily, low-dose aspirin also turns out to reduce risks of two serious diseases of the digestive tract: colon cancer and esophageal cancer. All of these benefits (and probably more) are the result of aspirin's effect on the synthesis and deployment of prostaglandins, suggesting, I think, how great their influence is on our health and well-being.

Like other control systems in the body, prostaglandins have ambivalent actions—for instance, they can both intensify or diminish inflammation and increase or decrease the clotting tendency of the blood. In order for the body to stay healthy, these two potentials must be properly balanced. If you are injured, you need the inflammatory response as a component of healing: Inflammation brings blood and immune cells to the injured area. Once that phase of healing is complete, it is important that inflammation not continue.

There are many different prostaglandins in several different families, each with different actions, but here is a simplifying principle: In general, prostaglandins derived from omega-6 fatty acids promote cell proliferation, inflammation, and blood clotting, while those derived from omega-3 fatty acids oppose those effects. Again, both are necessary and must work together in concert to maintain health. Too few of the former would impair cell growth and differentiation, increase risk of bleeding, and result in failure to mount adequate immune responses. Too few of the latter might increase risks of cancer, blood clots, and inflammatory and autoimmune diseases.

Mounting evidence suggests that dietary intake of EFAs can affect this balance. Even if LNA, an omega-3, is present in the diet, a high omega-6 to omega-3 ratio blocks production of the inhibitory prostaglandins. It is certain that the modern Western diet is seriously deficient in omega-3 EFAs. Moreover, that diet now provides a great excess of omega-6 EFAs, mainly in polyunsaturated vegetable oils and products made from them, creating an omega-6 to omega-3 ratio vastly different from what most people enjoyed in the past.

Widespread use of polyunsaturated vegetable oils is a dietary change that came with the twentieth century. So is the modern practice of eating meat from animals raised on grains devoid of omega-3 EFAs instead of grasses containing them. Therefore, it is more than possible that the epidemic of coronary heart disease and fatal heart attacks that took place in the twentieth century correlates not so much with any excesses in what people were consuming, but rather with deficiencies of protective factors that in the past neutralized the harmful effects of eating a lot of saturated fat and high-glycemic-index carbohydrates.

In April 1999 the National Institutes of Health convened a workshop on the Essentiality and Recommended Dietary Intakes for Omega-6 and Omega-3 Fatty Acids. Consensus was reached on the importance of reducing intake of the former, even as efforts are made to increase intake of the latter, for all people, including newborns. Participants felt this dietary change was critical to achieve optimal brain and cardiovascular function.

An earlier NIH meeting in September 1998 focused on the importance of omega-3 fatty acids in protecting the nervous system and promoting mental health. Of particular interest here is another of the longer-chain fatty acids in the omega-3 series, DHA, a component of fish oil. The body can make this from LNA, but, again, if the diet is top-heavy in omega-6 fatty acids, those will compete for a necessary enzyme, blocking synthesis of DHA. (For this reason, it might be advisable to eat fish and get the needed fatty acid preformed rather than relying on vegetarian sources of LNA like flax seeds and canola oil. I'll give you specific recommendations at the end of this section.) DHA is the main structural component of cell membranes in the brain. If it is deficient in the body, especially during late fetal development and early infant life, weakened architecture of the central nervous system may result, impairing learning ability, intelligence, and other aspects of mental function.

Some scientists are now lobbying for supplementation of infant formulas with DHA, and informed obstetricians advise pregnant women to eat salmon and sardines, especially in the last trimester and while breastfeeding. Other researchers are exploring the connection between omega-3 fatty acid deficiency and such conditions as autism, attention deficit disorder, and depression. Yet another possibility is that brains deficient in DHA are more susceptible to toxic injury that may result in degenerative diseases of later life such as Parkinson's disease, ALS (amyotrophic lateral sclerosis, Lou Gehrig's disease), and Alzheimer's disease. Watch for developments on all these fronts; they are exciting areas of ongoing research on dietary influences on health.

Some pages back I wrote that, beginning in the 1950s, doctors and nutritionists began urging people to eat polyunsaturated vegetable oils as "antidotes" to saturated fat and its unhealthy effect on LDL cholesterol. Most people who follow this advice—who replace butter with safflower oil or corn oil margarine—will see reductions in LDL cholesterol, but we now know that polyunsaturated oils also lower HDL cholesterol, the desirable fraction that represents the body's effort to remove cholesterol from tissues and blood and take it to the liver for elimination. So you now know of two problems associated with these oils: They lower good cholesterol along with bad, and they are the major cause of the unhealthy omega-6 to omega-3 ratio in our diets.

But there is more. The double bonds that characterize PUFAs are points of strain in fatty acid molecules, susceptible to attack by oxygen. When oxygen reacts with unsaturated fatty acids, the result is the formation of a range of dangerous compounds. Oxidized fat smells bad and tastes bad; it accounts for rancidity of fats and oils, of foods containing them (like nuts) and products made from them (chips, baked goods). The more double bonds a fatty acid contains, the higher the percentage of PUFAs in a given fat or oil, the greater the exposure to light, heat, and air—the greater the tendency toward oxidation and rancidity.

Flax oil—an excellent source of LNA as well as LA—is so unsaturated and therefore so reactive that it oxidizes very quickly on exposure to air, even at room temperature, becoming thicker and harder as it does. Under the name linseed oil it is the basis of oil paints and furniture finishes, because it goes on in liquid form, then "dries" to a hard finish. (Safflower oil used to be classified as a drying oil rather than an edible oil because its degree of unsaturation renders it almost as susceptible to rapid oxidation.) If you are unsure what rancid fat smells like, just sniff some linseed oil or oil paint, and if you detect anything similar in nuts, chips, flour, or baked goods you are tempted to eat, throw them out at once. Oxidized oils promote arterial damage, cancer, inflammation, degenerative disease, and premature aging of cells and tissues.

How they do so involves the generation of free radicals, highly reactive molecules that can initiate chain reactions of chemical disruption, injuring cell membranes, enzymes, and DNA itself. Such calamities are one variety of "oxidative stress" that our bodies must defend themselves against. They do so by relying on antioxidants, compounds that quench free radicals and neutralize destructive oxidation reactions. I'll have more to say about antioxidants when I discuss micronutrients; even though they abound in fresh fruits and vegetables, there may be reason to add them to the diet in supplemental form for extra protection.

Here is a simple experiment you can do in your kitchen to observe the relative tendencies of different kinds of fat to oxidize. Put small amounts of clarified butter, olive oil, and safflower oil in separate open containers and let them sit. Each day, sniff the containers and note when you can detect the telltale odor of rancidity. You will get it very soon with the safflower oil (mostly PUFAs), not so soon with the olive oil (mostly MUFAs, not many PUFAs), and very late with the clarified butter (mostly SFAs, few PUFAs). At higher temperatures and with greater exposure to light, the changes would take place faster.

When you deep-fry foods, the fat you use reaches very high temperatures. It would be a good idea not to reuse that fat. At least, it would be a good idea from the perspective of health; economically, it might not make sense, because fats and oils are costly. If you were a manufacturer of potato chips, the manager of an institutional cafeteria, or the owner of a restaurant, you could not afford to change the fat in your deep fryers after every use or even very frequently. You would reuse it and continue to reuse it until it imparted a bad taste to foods—that is, until oxidized fat reached levels at which its taste and smell could not be ignored.

A recent research paper in the *Journal of the American College of Cardiology* makes the possible consequences of this situation all too clear. Australian investigators fed volunteer subjects three different meals containing measured portions of fat. The first meal had 64.4 grams of used fat taken from the deep fryer of a fast-food restaurant. The second meal had the same amount of unused cooking fat, and the third was a low-fat meal (18.4 grams of fat). Four hours after a meal, the researchers used a noninvasive test to measure blood flow through the brachial artery, the main artery supplying the arm. They found significant restriction of blood flow in subjects following the first meal but not after the other two meals. Their interpretation of the finding was immediate dysfunction of the lining of the artery caused by oxidative stress resulting from entry into the blood of toxic compounds in the used fat. Think about that the next time you are tempted to eat fast food or order anything deep-fried in a restaurant.

If the propensity of polyunsaturated vegetable oils to oxidize into compounds that damage the cardiovascular system and promote cancer is not enough to convince you to limit your intake of them, let me tell you of a final and possibly greater danger they pose to health. I have said that a double bond in a fatty acid molecule strains it, forcing it to assume a shape other than a straight chain. Let's look at oleic acid, the most common MUFA and the principal fatty acid in olive oil. It is a nonessential, monounsaturated fatty acid. Two possibilities exist for the shape of oleic acid. Without going into unnecessary details, I will tell you that one shape is called the *cis* configuration, and the other the *trans* configuration. Because it takes a bit more energy to make *cis*-oleic acid than to make *trans*-oleic acid, *cis*-oleic acid has a tendency to assume the more stable *trans* form, but *trans*-oleic acid is unlikely to switch into the *cis* form.

Now, almost all natural fatty acids with double bonds (MUFAs and PUFAs) are *cis*-fatty acids, and since you know that PUFAs are important structural components of membranes and building blocks for very important hormones, you can also understand that the configuration of these molecules would determine how well they function in those roles. The body uses *cis* forms to build membranes and hormones; given *trans* forms to work with, it might produce defective membranes and defective hormones.

This is exactly the possibility that some medical experts say exists because of the way that food processors handle the vegetable oils that end up on our tables and in our bodies. Most vegetable oils you buy in the supermarket are extracted from hard seeds with heat, pressure, and chemical solvents. Such extraction methods supply more than enough opportunities to turn *cis*-fatty acids into their *trans* counterparts. *Trans*-fatty acids, or TFAs, are unnatural forms of unsaturated fatty acids that some experts call "funny fats." It is not funny that commercially processed oils are full of them. TFAs also form when oils suffer undue exposure to heat and light after extraction. And they are created in abundance when oils are subjected to a most unnatural process called partial hydrogenation.

Read the labels of almost any brands of cookies, crackers, other baked goods, or snack foods you pick up in the supermarket and you will find "partially hydrogenated oil" high on the list of ingredients. Often the particular oil or oils are specified: "partially hydrogenated soybean oil" or "partially hydrogenated cottonseed, soybean, and/or corn oil." These are still other examples of foodstuffs that humans never ate before the twentieth century, and I consider them chief suspects in undermining our health.

The purpose of hydrogenating oils is to harden them to improve their spreadability, mouth feel, baking qualities, and, especially, to extend the shelf life of products made from them, since more-saturated fats oxidize—go rancid—less quickly than less-saturated fats. To hydrogenate an oil, manufacturers heat it to high temperatures 120°–210°C or 248°–410°F with hydrogen gas under pressure in the presence of metal catalysts (usually nickel, sometimes platinum) for six to eight hours. If they carry this process out to completion, all double bonds break; the product will then contain neither *cis* nor *trans* forms of fatty acids, only straight-chain SFAs. But usually the process is stopped before completion, resulting in a complex mixture of compounds, including TFAs.

Margarine is made in this way, and its high content of TFAs—as high as 30 or 40 percent—is a principal reason I do not recommend it for consumption. Margarine has a colorful history, going back to the late 1860s, when, in the wake of a devastating cattle plague that drove butter prices sky high, the French Academy issued a call to develop a butter substitute. Originally made from blubber and spoiled milk, margarine became much more practical (and palatable) after 1900, when food technologists learned to partially hydrogenate liquid vegetable oils. Manufacturers could then source the cheapest oils throughout the world and turn them into an edible spread.

Through the 1920s and 1930s margarine makers worked steadily to improve the product's taste and appearance, and as they did so, its popularity increased. Margarine's only virtue in this period was its price: It was a cheap substitute for butter. Nonetheless, its market share grew to the point where the butter industry was threatened enough to take action. By midcentury the butter lobby was successful in getting laws enacted to thwart sales of the ersatz product. In America, margarine had to be sold uncolored, so that it resembled lard. It came with a capsule of yellow food coloring to be kneaded in by the housewife, often resulting in a bizarre-looking, streaked mass. Canadian law required margarine to be colored bright pink. Clever though they were, these measures failed to halt the growth of margarine sales.

Then, in the 1950s came the perceptual change that rocketed margarine ahead of butter in usage and kept it there. Instead of seeing margarine as a cheap substitute, consumers began buying it as a healthy alternative to butter. This was the direct result of doctors and nutritionists proclaiming that saturated fats were bad and vegetable oils good. To this day, when I look in the refrigerators of physicians of my generation and older I am more likely to find margarine there than butter. But, in fact, margarine is not a healthy alternative to anything. It is a highly processed food full of funny fats that cannot be good for us. The only question is how bad they are.

It is clear that *trans*-fatty acids are bad for hearts and arteries. They drive up production of cholesterol like SFAs and promote atherosclerosis, undoing any benefits the oils might have provided. I am certain that TFAs will eventually be found to be detrimental to health in many other ways as a result of their effects on membrane and hormone function. I believe they promote the development of cancer and degenerative disease, increase inflammation, accelerate aging, and obstruct immunity and healing. Therefore, I make a scrupulous attempt to keep them out of my diet, and I urge you to do the same. In practice that means avoiding margarine, vegetable shortening, and all products made with them or with partially hydrogenated oils of any kind. When you start reading labels to look for those sources of TFAs, you will be amazed and discouraged to see how prevalent they are in commercial foods. This recently got easier. In November 1999 the Food and Drug Administration began requiring that food labels list content of *trans*-fatty acids.

So this is what we've established with regard to fat: Too much saturated fat in the diet drives up bad cholesterol; therefore, unless you are confident of your Methuselah lineage, you should not eat much animal fat, especially butterfat (as in cheese and other whole-milk products), which is the main source of saturated fatty acids in the Western diet. You should also minimize consumption of the two "tropical oils," palm and coconut, which also contain high proportions of SFAs, saturated fats. Of the two, coconut is the worse. (If you like Thai or other curries made with coconut milk, try preparing them at home, substituting cashew milk, which is primarily monounsaturated fat. See page 121 for the recipe.) Some years ago, a vocal public outcry succeeded in having tropical oils removed from commercial food products. Ironically, manufacturers replaced them with partially hydrogenated oils, which are even worse. Polyunsaturated vegetable oils lower good cholesterol along with bad, worsen an already unhealthy omega-6 to omega-3 ratio of essential fatty acids, are too susceptible to oxidation, and are likely to contain harmful TFAs as a result of processing. Margarine is out, as are all foods containing partially hydrogenated oils.

What we should be eating instead are the monounsaturated oils and fats and oils rich in omega-3 essential fatty acids, and these should be the main fats in the optimum diet. Monounsaturated fat lowers LDL cholesterol without disturbing HDL, resists oxidation much more than polyunsaturated oils, and is used by the body as a source of caloric energy almost as efficiently as saturated fat.

These good fats have various sources. Many nuts contain primarily monounsaturated oils, among them cashews, pistachios, and macadamias. Walnuts are especially valuable as a source of omega-3 fatty acids in the form of LNA. Shunned by advocates of spartan, low-fat regimens, nuts turn out to be healthy additions to the diet, much to my delight, since I have always enjoyed eating them. Recent studies suggest that eating a portion (say, a small handful) of nuts a day can lower LDL cholesterol and reduce serum triglycerides. Nuts are also a good source of fiber, minerals, and vitamin E. I recommend buying raw, natural, unsalted nuts and keeping them in the refrigerator until needed to protect them from going rancid. Once nuts are roasted or chopped, the oils in them will oxidize quickly. If you like cooked nuts, you can dry-roast them yourself in the oven or toss them about in a hot skillet. Do not store them for long after heating them.

Nut oils are flavorful, but because they have a high PUFA content, they are very susceptible to oxidation and should never be heated. Use walnut oil or hazelnut oil sparingly in salad dressings and keep them away from light and heat. Nut butters are also great in moderation. Look for almond, cashew, and macadamia-nut butters as healthy alternatives to peanut butter, which has a higher percentage of saturated fat and is likely to contain traces of aflatoxin, a potent, natural carcinogen produced by a mold that commonly grows on peanuts. In addition, many commercial brands of peanut butter contain partially hydrogenated oils—read labels!

Pumpkin seeds are an omega-3 source and make a pleasant snack. I buy raw, organic ones, keep them refrigerated, and eat them frequently. If you like them toasted, cook small quantities in a dry skillet and use them up quickly. It is possible to find dark green pumpkin-seed oil in natural food stores. Take the usual precautions with it, and use it only in cold dishes.

Avocados, another no-no on low-fat diets, are full of monounsaturated fat. You can make a butter alternative by mashing a ripe avocado and seasoning it to taste. Try it as a spread on bread to replace some of the saturated fat in your diet with a healthier form. You can find avocado oil in natural food stores, but it is bland and expensive and adds nothing special to dishes made with it.

By contrast, olive oil is highly flavored and adds a great deal to food. It has the highest percentage of monounsaturated fat of any of the edible oils (77 percent), and high-quality brands are now available in ordinary supermarkets. Because ripe olives are soft fruits rather than hard seeds, their fat can be extracted without using the harsh methods necessary to produce most vegetable oils. The best olive oil, labeled "extra-virgin," comes from the first, gentle pressing of the fruits. Professional chefs often tell us to save it for special uses, like dipping bread in it at the table or dressing salads, and to use lower-quality forms for cooking. I disagree. All the oil you eat should be the highest quality obtainable to minimize consumption of oxidized fat and *trans*-fatty acids. Delicious, organic, extra-virgin olive oil from California and Italy is now easy to find. Experiment with different brands to become familiar with the range of flavors of this useful oil.

The main disadvantage of olive oil is that it provides almost none of the essential fatty acids, no LNA and hardly any LA, but that just means that if you make olive oil your principal dietary fat, as I recommend that you do, you must make sure you are taking in an adequate amount of omega-3s from other sources. Some people find the flavor of olive oil too strong or inappropriate for certain dishes, such as Asian stir fries and cookies. One possibility is to use "light" olive oil for these recipes. It has a light color and neutral flavor, but the refining process that has removed color and flavor probably also reduces its health benefits.

Another possibility is to use canola oil, the modern version of rapeseed oil, a traditional cooking fat of India and southern China. Rape is in the mustard family, and its seed contains some omega-3s in the form of LNA, along with a substantial amount of monounsaturated fat—62 percent of the total. Unfortunately, canola oil also contains up to 5 percent of erucic acid, a toxic fatty acid, which to my mind cancels out its potential value as an omega-3 source. (The omega-3 fraction may even be removed from much commercial canola oil, because it decreases shelf life of the product.) Canola oil is neutral flavored, widely available, and heavily promoted as a healthy, monounsaturated fat, but I consider it a distant runner-up to olive oil and use it rarely. Commercial canola oil is extracted in ways (heat, solvents, bleaching) that damage the oil, and pesticides are used heavily on rape. If you do use canola oil, buy organic, expeller-pressed brands available in health food stores or natural food sections of supermarkets.

The only other vegetable oil with predominately monounsaturated fat (49 percent) is peanut oil, which also has a neutral taste. It contains some omega-6 fatty acids but no omega-3s, along with more SFAs than canola oil and more PUFAs than olive oil. I don't recommend it because methods of extraction damage its unsaturated fat content. Besides, like peanut butter, it may contain traces of aflatoxin.

Two special oils that are becoming more available are flax oil and hemp oil, both excellent sources of omega-3s. Flax seeds are the richest vegetable source of LNA, but the oil expressed from them is so high in PUFAs (72 percent) that it is very susceptible to damage. Freshly pressed flax oil is sweet and nutty; however, by the time it gets to your table, it is likely to have an unmistakable undertone of oil paint. Look for flax oil in small, opaque bottles in refrigerated cases or freezers of natural food stores. Don't use any that tastes like linseed oil. Keep it refrigerated, never heat it, and use it up quickly once you open the bottle. You can use flax oil in salad dressing or add it to other cold dishes.

Hemp is the plant (*Cannabis sativa*) that produces marijuana, but it is at least as well known throughout the world as a source of high-quality fiber and edible seeds and oil. Hemp oil is greenish, also with a delicious, nutty flavor, and is also an excellent source of essential fatty acids, although it provides less LNA (omega-3) and more LA (omega-6) than flax oil. A major problem is that hemp is illegal. Even though the seeds and oil contain no intoxicating properties, their production for food is limited by restrictions on growers, and the quality of edible hemp products is therefore compromised. Nonetheless, I have started to see some good-quality hemp oil in natural food stores. It is sold like flax oil and should be used in the same way.

Nature protects these delicate oils from oxidation by enclosing them in tough seed coats. My preference is to eat the seeds to take advantage of their omega-3s rather than bothering with the extracted oils. Flax seeds are very cheap—you can buy them in bulk in natural food stores—and they keep well in storage. (I would still store them in the refrigerator.) If you eat them whole, they will pass through you undigested; you must grind them to get their EFAs. I suggest buying an electric coffee grinder that you dedicate to flax. Grind the seeds— say half a cup at a time—to a coarse meal and sprinkle it on food such as cereal, salad, baked potatoes, or other vegetables. You will find it has a pleasant, nutty taste. You can also buy ready-ground flax meal, but that defeats the purpose. Once ground, with greatly increased surface area, flax seeds are especially susceptible to oxidative damage. Be aware that flax seeds, as opposed to flax oil, contain a great deal of fiber that will increase stool bulk and even act as a laxative depending on how much you eat. (Flax seeds also contain phytoestrogens, protective compounds I will tell you about when I discuss micronutrients.) Two tablespoons of freshly ground flax seeds daily will add a good measure of omega-3 fatty acids to your diet.

In the case of hemp seeds, I prefer to dry-toast them and eat them as a snack. Put a layer of raw hemp seeds in a dry skillet and stir them over medium high heat until they begin to pop and lightly brown. Add a tiny amount of olive oil to coat them, remove them from the heat, and season them to taste—for example, with salt, soy sauce, garlic powder, or chile powder. Let them cool before eating them. They are quite delicious. Use them up quickly, which should not be a problem.

I mentioned above that soy oil, a predominately polyunsaturated oil, also provides EFAs, as do mayonnaise and commercial salad dressings made with soy oil and canola oil. Egg yolks in mayonnaise may also contribute, although probably mostly omega-6s, unless the chickens were lucky enough to be free ranging or received supplemental algae in their feed. If you use mayonnaise and bottled salad dressings, you would do well to look for natural brands containing those oils. I am a great proponent of eating soybeans and foods made from them for many reasons, one being the content of EFAs in the oil, but I do not recommend soy oil for cooking, because the extraction of it involves heat, solvents, bleaches, and other treatments that damage its high content of PUFAs.

That brings us to the fish oils, perhaps the most valuable sources of omega-3s, certainly of the preformed, very long chain omega-3s, EPA and DHA, that appear to be critically important for optimum cardio-vascular, neurological, and mental health. Let me repeat that our bodies can make these vital nutrients from dietary LNA, but that the conversion is often inefficient, especially if the necessary enzymes are overwhelmed by excess omega-6 fatty acids in the diet. For that reason, I think it is useful to eat the oily, cold-water fish that provide them, such as salmon, sardines, mackerel, and herring. The fat of cold-water marine mammals such as seals and whales is also full of them—and is surely the reason that traditional Inuit did not suffer from atherosclerosis and coronary heart disease, despite their consumption of huge amounts of total fat and saturated fat.

(Inuit today definitely suffer. For one thing, the fat of marine mammals now contains high levels of toxins, including pesticides and industrial pollutants that have found their way into the oceans. Even though Inuit live in relatively pristine areas of the world, like Greenland, their own body fat and breast milk are now full of worrisome toxins. This sad situation illustrates the principle that large animals, living at the top of food chains, concentrate environmental toxins in their fat. It is also a remarkable indictment of the environmental policies of all nations. Furthermore, many Inuit now have incorporated some of the worst offerings of the modern food industry into their diets, including processed vegetable fats. Consider, for example, what has happened to "Eskimo ice cream," a traditional summertime treat of seal fat mixed with berries. The contemporary version is a bowl of vegetable shortening, stirred together with sugar and fruit.)

Marine mammals are not in our diets, but fish certainly are. I will discuss them in more detail, pointing out their advantages and disadvantages, in the next section on protein. Here I will simply repeat that it is good to include fatty fish in the diet; I recommend two to three servings of them a week, more if possible. Generally, I do not recommend taking extracted fish oils in supplemental form. In the first place, if you are trying to keep total fat intake to moderate levels, it seems a shame to waste your fat calories on capsules. Second, fish oils, since they are so unsaturated, oxidize quickly. They are likely to be more intact in fish than in supplements. Third, a serious problem with fish is toxic contamination—I will say more about that in the next section, too—which is why I am concerned about commercial fish-oil supplements. I would need assurance that they are free of the toxins that are so prevalent in fish today.

Now, having armed you with a great deal of information about dietary fats, the dangers of bad fats, and the benefits and sources of good fats, I would like to conclude this section by summarizing my views on these most important macronutrients and giving specific recommendations about using them.

• One outstanding danger of very low fat diets (10 to 20 percent of calories as fat) is essential fatty acid deficiency. The danger is greater on vegetarian low-fat diets, since they exclude fish and eggs and include seeds and oils that worsen an already distorted omega-6 to omega-3 ratio. Unless great care is taken to get enough omega-3 fatty acids on these diets, all the health risks associated with deficiency of them will rise.

• The second danger of very low fat diets is increased cardiovascular risks due to excess consumption of carbohydrates and attendant changes in the serum lipid profile. In general, fat and carbohydrate substitute for each other in the diet: Lower one and the other increases. Some people eating 10 percent of calories as fat eat 70 or even 80 percent of calories as carbohydrate—way too much—and develop high levels of serum triglycerides. In addition, men on these diets show decreased amounts of HDL along with abnormal LDL particles, which are smaller and denser, a form that may be linked to a high risk of atherosclerosis.

• These risks may be overshadowed by a large decrease in overall LDL, which may account in part for Dr. Ornish's ability to demonstrate reversal of coronary artery disease with his program of lifestyle modification that combines very low fat diet with moderate exercise and intensive group support. I have no hesitation about referring patients with existing cardiac disease to this program and others like it, especially patients facing unappealing allopathic interventions like coronary artery bypass graft surgery or angioplasty. They certainly have the motivation to undertake such a rigid diet, and these programs reduce the occurrence of so-called cardiac events—heart attacks, and the like—in patients with diseased hearts. But I wonder if disease reversal takes place in spite of the diet or whether a more palatable diet with the right kinds of fat, combined with the same sort of exercise and group support, would work even better.

• Palatability of food decreases sharply as fat calories drop below 20 percent of total calories. Maintaining a 10-percent-fat diet is very difficult unless you live at a spa, hire a professional chef, or are willing to give up the pleasure of eating.

• Most people can enjoy optimum health on a diet containing 30 percent fat. The example of Crete and other Mediterranean regions suggests that even more fat in the diet might be acceptable, as long as it is made up of predominately monounsaturated and essential fatty acids, with a favorable (i.e., low) omega-6 to omega-3 ratio.

• Reduce the amount of saturated fat in the diet by cutting back on butter, cream, whole milk, yogurt, and, especially, cheese made from whole milk. If you like dairy products, try to use low-fat forms, such as low-fat or skim milk, and cheese made from part-skim milk. Cut back on meat and unskinned poultry or substitute wild game. Minimize consumption of palm and coconut oils. Conventional nutritionists recommend an equal distribution of the three kinds of fat, so that in a 30-percent-fat diet, 10 percent of the calories would come from saturated fat, 10 from monounsaturated fat, and 10 from polyunsaturated fat. I recommend a ratio of 1:2:1—that is, 5 percent of calories from saturated fat, 20 from monounsaturated fat, and 5 from polyunsaturated fat. If you are eating 2,000 calories a day, 30 percent of those calories—600—can come from fat, and no more than 100 should be from saturated fat. The more saturated fat you eat, the more important it is to pay attention to essential fatty acid intake and the omega-6 to omega-3 ratio.

• Avoid polyunsaturated vegetable oils (safflower, sunflower, sesame, corn, soy, cottonseed) and products made from them.

• Strictly avoid margarine and vegetable shortening and products made from them.

• Strictly avoid all products containing partially hydrogenated oils of any kind.

• Use extra-virgin olive oil as your main fat. If you do not want a strong flavor of olive oil in a particular dish, search out milder-flavored brands or use a light olive oil.

• Organic, expeller-pressed canola oil may be used in moderation as an alternative, neutral-tasting oil.

• Buy all oils in smaller rather than larger sizes and use them up quickly once you open them. Protect all oils from light and heat. If you use olive oil frequently, keep a small amount out and refrigerate the rest. It will slowly congeal in the cold due to its 14 percent content of SFAs. Hardened olive oil is easily returned to the liquid state by placing its bottle in warm water.

• Flavorful nut oils (walnut, hazelnut, pistachio) may be used in moderation in cold foods.

• Roasted (dark) sesame oil is another oil that is acceptable in the small quantities used to flavor Chinese and Japanese recipes. Its flavor is quite concentrated; a teaspoon or two is enough for most dishes.

• Pumpkin-seed oil, flax oil, and hemp oil are all rich in essential fatty acids, including the vital omega-3s, and can be used. Make sure they smell and taste good before you use them, protect them from light and heat, and use them up quickly in dressings or other cold foods. I am more in favor of eating the seeds they come from: raw or freshy toasted pumpkin and hemp seeds, and freshly ground flax meal.

• Never heat any oil to the point of smoking and never breathe the smoke of heated or burning fat—it is highly toxic.

• Do not eat deep-fried foods in restaurants, especially fast-food restaurants.

• If you deep-fry foods at home (which you are better off not doing much of), throw the oil out after cooking rather than saving it for reuse.

• You can spend some of your fat calories on avocados, nuts (not peanuts), and nut butters (not peanut butter). Walnuts are particularly valuable nutritionally, because they are an omega-3 source. Raw, natural nuts are best; if you like them roasted, cook them yourself and use them up quickly. Store nuts and nut butters in the refrigerator.

• If you eat eggs, use only eggs from free-range chickens, or look for the new eggs fortified with omega-3 fatty acids.

• If you use mayonnaise or bottled salad dressings, buy natural brands made with olive, soy, or canola oils.

• Eat soybeans and foods made from them (soymilk, tofu, mock meats) for their omega-3 fatty acids.

• Eat fish that contain omega-3s regularly, at least two to three times a week. If you do not eat fish, concentrate on the vegetable sources of omega-3s (walnuts, flax seeds, hemp seeds), and make an effort to decrease consumption of omega-6 fatty acids by cutting way down on the common vegetable oils, other than olive oil, and products made from them.

• It is especially important for pregnant women in the last trimester and nursing mothers to get adequate amounts of omega-3s, preferably from fish.

• If you like chocolate, you will be glad to know that the body handles cocoa butter like olive oil—i.e., cocoa butter does not raise cholesterol and has a beneficial effect on the serum lipid profile. Buy high-quality dark chocolate only. Milk chocolate contains butterfat, which moves cholesterol levels in the wrong direction, and cheaper products replace cocoa butter with undesirable fats like palm oil, which is highly saturated, or even with partially hydrogenated oils. Read labels!

I hope I have not overwhelmed you with information about fat. It is information you need to help you navigate through a confusing world and be a savvy consumer. The kind of fat you eat has a major influence on your health and longevity, and misinformation on this subject is the rule rather than the exception. Note that, as is the case with carbohydrates, it is the processing of fat-containing foods that reduces their protective qualities and makes them unhealthy—yet another reason to include more natural, unprocessed foods in your diet.

IV

PROTEIN REVISITED: HOW MUCH IS ENOUGH?

If you tell people you are a vegetarian, a usual response is, "Where are you getting your protein?" No one ever asks, "Where are you getting your fat?" or "Where are you getting your sugar?" It is only protein that people seem to worry about getting enough of. (A much more appropriate question, as you learned in the last chapter, would be, "Where are you getting your omega-3 fatty acids?") In the 1960s and 1970s, when large numbers of young Americans began experimenting with vegetarianism, conventional nutritionists warned them and their parents of the danger of protein deficiency, and one wrote in a syndicated newspaper column that it was impossible to maintain health on diets that excluded animal foods.

A popular book of the time—*Diet for a Small Planet* by Frances Moore Lappé—unintentionally reinforced this concern by explaining that animal protein was "complete," providing all of the ten essential amino acids, whereas vegetable protein was "incomplete," lacking one or more of them. The solution, the author suggested, was "protein combining"—eating grains and beans together, for example—so that the amino acid deficiencies of one food would be covered by another food at the same meal. She meant well and was actually arguing for vegetarian diets, pointing out that feeding grains to animals was incredibly wasteful, when those grains could be put to more efficient use feeding people. Unfortunately, all the talk about incomplete protein left vegetarians feeling vulnerable; unless they had calculators and tables of food composition at the ready, they could be on a fast track to malnutrition.

The collective consciousness is full of images of malnutrition in general and protein deficiency in particular, such as newspaper photographs of starving children in Africa with grotesquely swollen bellies. I think the emotions stimulated by these images resonate with a cultural bias common to societies dependent on agriculture. In most of them for most of history, rich people ate meat while poor people subsisted on carbohydrate staples—rice, potatoes, bread, and the like. In fact, the ability to put slabs of animal protein on the table regularly has been one of the most obvious signs of affluence of individuals and of the prosperity of nations. ("A chicken in every pot" was a classic political candidate's promise to voters.) The hunter-gatherer societies that preceded the rise of agriculture accorded highest status to those who were the most successful hunters. The man who brought back the most meat for the tribe would be a good candidate for tribal leader.

Thus our attitudes toward protein are shaped by a variety of historical, cultural, and economic factors and are strongly influenced by the media. Protein *is* special in the sense that it contains nitrogen, is made up of very complex molecules, and gives organisms their biochemical identity. Protein foods of animal origin are perishable and expensive. From the point of view of general nutrition, however, protein is neither more nor less special or desirable than fat and carbohydrate. The body needs all three of the macronutrients in proper balance, and deficiencies of any of them are impediments to optimum health.

Research has discredited the idea that vegetable protein is incomplete and therefore less valuable than animal protein. The body is clever enough to find missing essential amino acids if a meal does not contain them all. It can get them from the vast numbers of bacteria that inhabit the lower intestinal tract or from the vast numbers of cells that slough off the lining of the digestive tract every day. Not only can vegetarians survive and be healthy, studies consistently show them to be healthier and longer-lived than meat eaters, although whether this is due to what they don't eat, what they do eat, or other aspects of lifestyle is not clear.

In fact, protein needs are much lower than most people imagine, and the risk of protein deficiency for most of us is negligible. The early signs of protein deficiency are clear: hair and nails stop growing, and wounds do not heal. I often recommend low-protein diets to patients with allergies, as well as those with autoimmunity, liver, or kidney problems, and I have never seen these symptoms appear in any of them. Even athletes, persons doing heavy physical labor, and pregnant women are not at greater risk; ordinary diets supply more than enough protein for them. Protein needs are increased in nursing mothers, actively growing children, and persons recovering from serious illness and injury, but even in those cases ordinary diets are usually fine. Only people experimenting with strange, very restrictive diets—fruitarians, for example—or alcoholics or very poor people subsisting on starch are likely to become protein deficient in our societies.

Having said that, I must also say at the start of this discussion that I think we know less about protein than we do about carbohydrate and fat, particularly about individual variations in needs for it and for specific amino acids. Some individuals who eliminate animal protein from their diet find themselves moping and drooping; they feel better instantly when they again eat meat. Others say that soy foods and grain burgers suit them just fine. Some people seem to do best eating protein as the main course of every meal. Others feel lethargic if they eat too much protein at even one meal. So finding the right amount of this macronutrient to include in the optimum diet is tricky.

I recommend getting 50 to 60 percent of calories from carbohydrate, as much of that as possible from unrefined low-glycemic-index carbohydrate foods, and 30 percent of calories from fat, mostly from monounsaturated oils and foods high in omega-3 fatty acids. That leaves 10 to 20 percent of calories from protein, which, on a 2,000-calorie daily diet would be 200 to 400 calories or about 50 to 100 grams. Advocates of low-fat, high-carbohydrate diets would say that 20 percent protein is too much, while those in favor of low-carbohydrate, high-protein diets would say it is not enough. I think 10 to 20 percent of calories as protein is the right general range.

Recall that protein consumed in excess of the body's needs for growth becomes fuel that the body burns for energy, and that protein is a relatively inefficient and dirty fuel compared to carbohydrate and fat. Because protein molecules are so complex, the ratio of energy expended to energy gained in dismantling and metabolizing them is less favorable than that for running the metabolic engine on fat or carbohydrate. (This may be a reason why many people find high-protein diets help them lose weight.) Because protein molecules contain nitrogen, when they are burned to yield energy they leave nitrogenous residues instead of just producing water and carbon dioxide, the only waste products of the metabolism of fat and carbohydrate.

As I said earlier, the end waste product of the metabolic combustion of protein is the simple compound ammonia. To protect itself from this very toxic substance, the body converts it to urea, a task that falls on the liver. Urea is much less toxic than ammonia, but still a waste product of metabolism that must be eliminated. It is up to the kidneys to remove it from the bloodstream and get it out of the system in urine. High-protein diets, therefore, in which much of the protein consumed winds up as fuel for energy production, have the following effects on the body: 1) an increased workload on the liver, 2) an increased workload on the kidneys, and 3) possible exposure of sensitive organs to toxic metabolic wastes. These consequences deserve closer scrutiny.

In liver failure, which can result from destruction of liver tissue by cancer, by infection (chronic hepatitis), or by inflammation (alcoholic cirrhosis), the immediate relationship between dietary protein and ammonia in the blood is obvious. Doctors routinely measure blood ammonia levels of hospitalized patients in liver failure as a sensitive indicator of their progress or lack of it. As blood ammonia rises, brain function declines, eventually producing loss of consciousness (hepatic coma) and death. It is easy to detect the odor of ammonia on the breath of a patient in or near hepatic coma. It is also easy to accelerate or retard the development of this medical catastrophe by increasing or decreasing the patient's intake of protein. Unfortunately, in my experience, patients with early-stage liver disease rarely get the important advice to cut down on dietary protein as a way to reduce the workload on that organ.

Similarly, in end-stage kidney disease, when patients must go on blood dialysis or begin preparing for kidney transplant operations, doctors warn them not to eat too much protein. If the patients had started following this recommendation years before, they might have postponed the need for drastic medical and surgical interventions. The indicator for kidney function is measurement of blood urea nitrogen (BUN); a rise from normal low levels correlates with an inability of the kidneys to clear the urea made by the liver in its effort to detoxify the metabolic waste of protein metabolism.

Increased production of urea not only taxes the kidneys, it requires diuresis—an increase of water loss in urine—to flush the compound out of the body. One not-so-obvious consequence of the diuretic effect of a high-protein diet is accompanying loss of minerals, especially calcium. It is well known that high-protein diets promote calcium loss and so increase the risk of osteoporosis, the common condition of weakened bones that affects many older people, diminishing their stature, deforming their spines, and increasing their risk of fractures, especially of hips.

Most people think that eating a lot of protein, animal protein especially, builds strong bodies and bones. That may not be the case. Women in sub-Saharan Africa have very strong bones, even though they eat grain-based diets and get only a small fraction (about 250 milligrams a day) of the recommended intake of calcium (1,500 milligrams a day). On the other hand, traditional Inuit, who eat huge amounts of animal protein along with their fat, have severe osteoporosis. (Of course, genetics and vitamin D levels also differ in these populations. The body makes vitamin D, necessary for absorption and utilization of calcium, from cholesterol on exposure to sunlight, and Inuit get little sun in the winter. Nonetheless, I think very different levels of protein intake in these disparate populations strongly influence the condition of their bones.)

A further possibility is that high-protein diets may irritate the immune system, keeping it off-balance and making it more likely to react against harmless substances in the environment like pollen and animal dander (allergy) or to attack the body's own tissues (autoimmunity). Allergy and autoimmunity both have significant genetic roots and both are also influenced by environmental triggers. For example, the protein in cow's milk—casein—seems to be the responsible environmental trigger that sets off common forms of allergy in infants and young children and possibly autoimmune reactions as well. The timing of first exposure to milk protein may be all-important. If one or both parents has an allergic history, a child is at increased risk to develop allergy as well. Exposing the child to milk protein too early in life—before the age of two, say—may activate the allergic potential, causing such reactions as eczema (allergic dermatitis) and asthma, and setting up the immune system for high allergic responsiveness for the rest of the child's life. If cow's milk is withheld until the critical period has passed, allergy may not develop.

Research also suggests that during some critical window of early life, cow's milk protein may also trigger the autoimmune reaction that destroys insulin-producing cells of the pancreas, actualizing an inherited tendency toward the development of juvenile diabetes. In practice I find that patients with problems of allergy and autoimmunity often improve on low-protein diets, especially on plant-based diets that restrict animal protein in general and milk protein in particular. Since the immune system focuses primarily on protein molecules in determining whether a substance belongs in the body or not, it makes sense that one could quiet a sensitive immune system by not flooding the system with more dietary protein than it needs for growth, maintenance, and repair of tissues.

Let me repeat that there is much uncertainty here. We just do not know why some people do better eating more protein and others do better eating less, and research is definitely needed to document the health problems that may be associated with diets that supply a high percentage of calories as protein. There is also much confusion about the kinds of protein foods that should predominate in the diet for optimum health. At the risk of going beyond what we know scientifically at present, I would like to examine this question and give you my opinions, starting with a consideration of the relative advantages and disadvantages of animal versus nonanimal sources of protein.

Animal sources of protein include meat from cows, pigs, and sheep, and to a much lesser extent, of wild game like deer, elk, and moose; the flesh of chicken and other poultry; eggs, mostly from chickens; milk, mainly from cows, and products derived from it; fish, and shellfish.

Because we are much more closely related to animals than to plants, their proteins are more like ours, and it is easier for the human body to rearrange them into new molecules for its own needs. As energy sources, animal and plant proteins are equivalent; however, there are important differences between common animal and nonanimal protein foods in terms of what other elements they supply or fail to supply.

For example, meat, obtained mostly from the skeletal muscles of large herbivores, comes marbled with fat that is mostly saturated and makes a significant contribution to the total saturated fat intake of human carnivores. Most people prefer meat with a higher content of this internal fat, because it is juicier and more tender. In fact, in the grading system for beef used by the U.S. Department of Agriculture, the highest grade of "prime" goes to the meat with the most fat in it. Beef fat is the worst animal fat in terms of chemical composition, containing 51 percent saturated fatty acids (SFAs), 44 percent mono-unsaturated fatty acids (MUFAs), and only a trace of polyunsaturated fatty acids (PUFAs). By contrast, the fat of pigs—lard—has 41 percent SFAs, 47 percent MUFAs, and 12 percent PUFAs.

Americans' and others' (Argentineans' even more than Americans') love of beef not only helps push daily protein intake far above basic protein needs but also skews dietary fat in an unhealthy direction. Remember also that, although the PUFA content of fat of all domestic animals—pigs and sheep, as well as cows—includes some linoleic acid, it has no omega-3s as a result of the practice of fattening these animals on grains. Thus eating a lot of meat contributes to the present undesirable ratio of omega-6 to omega-3 fatty acids in the modern diet.

A famous restaurant in Amarillo, Texas, appropriately named the Big Texan Steak Ranch, serves a seventy-two-ounce steak, accompanied by a shrimp cocktail, baked potato, salad, and bread. If you finish the whole meal within an hour, you don't have to pay for it; otherwise, the cost is $50 plus tax. That is four and a half pounds of beef at one sitting, just over two kilograms. I called a manager of the restaurant for more details and was told that, on average, one person a day attempts this challenge, and one person in six succeeds. The "winners" have included a sixty-nine-year-old grandmother and an eleven-year-old boy, with the speed record held by a former pitcher for the Cincinnati Reds baseball team, who ate the whole meal in nine and a half minutes. Another record holder is a former pro wrestling star, Klondike Bill, who ate two of the meals in one hour.

An Argentinean mixed grill (*parrillada mixta*) is in almost the same category, providing astonishing portions of beef, along with sausages and organs of the cow, all grilled on an open fire. It is the fare of gauchos and comes with all of the romanticized machismo of cowboys throughout the Americas.

Doctors often warn patients away from organ meats—liver, kidneys, sweetbreads, and the like—because they are high in cholesterol; but as I have pointed out, cholesterol that you eat has far less impact on cholesterol in your blood than the saturated fat you eat. I am more concerned about possible concentrations of heavy metals, environmental toxins, and infectious agents in organ meats, which is the main reason I recommend avoiding them, even though they are sources of B vitamins and some trace minerals. The possibility of infection from animal organs, though small at the moment, came spectacularly to public attention with the outbreak of bovine spongiform encephalopathy —"mad cow disease"—in England in the late 1980s. Human cases of this fatal brain disease that resulted from eating the meat of infected cows are well documented; whether the meat included brain tissue or not is unclear. (Sloppy procedures in slaughterhouses can contaminate muscle tissue with bits of brain.)

This disease and variants of it that occur spontaneously in humans and many animals can be transmitted from one species to another by eating infected tissue. In England, the disease became widespread in beef cattle as a result of the unnatural practice of feeding them parts of carcasses of sheep (!) infected with scrapie, the ovine form of spongiform encephalopathy. The agents responsible for these diseases are prions, a newly recognized class of pathogens that carry information but are nonliving. Prions are simply very small proteins that can disrupt cellular information systems and are remarkably resistant to most of the methods of disinfection used to destroy more complex and familiar disease agents like viruses, bacteria, and parasites. They cause slowly developing, incurable brain degeneration that is always fatal, and their discovery has made scientists suddenly aware of hazards of animal products never before considered.

After studying prions and the diseases they cause, I have stopped using bone meal and blood meal in my garden; if animals that yielded the meal were infected, inhaling dust from these products could put prions in your system. I now recommend synthetic rather than animal-derived hormones to patients with endocrine deficiencies, and I am more comfortable than ever with my own lacto-pesco-vegetarian diet (milk products and fish in addition to plants). I do not cite the spongiform encephalopathies to scare you away from eating meat, but I do urge you never to eat brains. I also recommend not eating other organ meats frequently or in quantity, as the risk is much higher than with muscle.

Sloppiness in slaughterhouses can also contaminate meat with fecal matter and dangerous bacteria, especially the deadly forms of E. coli that have caused much publicized illness among meat eaters in both the United States and Japan.

Separate from the possibility of serious infections carried in meat is the issue of toxic contamination of foods of animal origin, having to do both with our methods of raising animals and with environmental contamination in general. Commercially raised animals are fed estrogenic hormones to make them gain weight faster and antibiotics to increase growth rates. Residues of these drugs in meat can impact human health adversely. The hormones add to total estrogenic pressure on women from many sources, increasing risk of breast cancer, other cancers of the female reproductive system, and other estrogenically driven conditions (fibrocystic changes in breasts and uterine fibroid tumors, for example). The hormones may also promote the development of prostate cancer in men. Antibiotics in meat certainly contribute to the escalating problem of antibiotic-resistant bacteria, which are becoming prevalent in the world.

Furthermore, large animals, even herbivorous ones, live at the tops of food chains, the sequences of organisms in which larger ones feed on smaller ones, which feed on smaller ones still, and so forth. At each higher level of a food chain, environmental toxins are more concentrated. From this point of view, diets lower in animal foods are definitely more healthful because they deliver lower doses of environmental toxins, a broad range of pollutants that can cause cancer and damage to many systems of the body, including the immune system and nervous system. (Recall the plight of traditional Inuit eating the meat and fat of large marine mammals.) I will return to this theme when I tell you about the pros and cons of eating fish and, in the following section, of conventional versus organic produce.

A small number of farmers specialize in producing more healthful meat from animals raised organically and certified to be free of hormones and antibiotics. Some of these animals spend all of their lives grazing in the wild rather than being fattened in feed lots and, as a result, are not only leaner but also have a much better profile of fatty acids in their fat. Other farmers are trying to popularize the meat of the American bison (buffalo) as a healthful alternative to beef. And some restaurants and specialty food suppliers offer the meat of wild game. Of course, all these products are expensive and not available on the mass market, but if you are a dedicated meat eater, you would do well to learn more about these alternative choices.

Poultry differs from the meat of large grazing animals in several important respects. For one thing, its fat is external to muscle instead of being distributed through it, so that it can be removed before cooking, a great advantage if you are trying to reduce consumption of saturated fat. (Also, there may be a higher concentration of pesticides and other environmental toxins in the fat of animals than in the muscles.) Chicken fat has a healthier composition than the fat of cows, pigs, and sheep—only 30 percent SFAs. Essential fatty acids are present, but, again, only omega-6s in the grain-fed, caged birds that dominate the market. Antibiotics and hormones are used in abundance in raising chickens for food, and a risk of infection exists as well, especially from *Salmonella* bacteria as a result of unsanitary methods of slaughter and butchering. Here, too, more healthful versions are available with some difficulty and at higher prices. Specialty stores sell organically raised, drug- and hormone-free chicken from birds that got to run around on the ground and scratch for food. If I ate chicken, it would be the only kind I would buy.

All of these considerations apply to other birds raised for food: turkeys, ducks, and geese. In recent years, lean turkey meat has appeared as a substitute for beef and pork in sausages, burgers, and other processed meats—better options because of their much lower content of saturated fat. Ducks and geese are fattier than chicken; if you eat them, you should take care to remove as much of their fat as possible before cooking.

I have already discussed eggs (of chickens) as good sources of omega-3 fatty acids if they come from free-range chickens or chickens whose diets are supplemented with omega-3-rich algae. It is the yolk of the egg that contains the fat (and the cholesterol); egg white is pure protein of a sort that the body can easily assimilate and use. If you like eggs and take care to cook them in healthful ways, you can include whole eggs from drug- and hormone-free, uncaged chickens in the optimum diet in moderation, say an average of one egg a day.

Before I leave the subject of flesh foods, I would like to mention two concerns about them that demand thoughtful consideration and personal decision. The first is the ethics of causing animals to suffer; the second is the ecological consequence of depending on animals for food. At the beginning of this book, I alluded to the existential dilemma of living at the expense of other life and noted that vegetarianism, although it may feel more comfortable, is not a way out. Nonetheless, if we eat organisms that are more like us, the problem becomes more difficult to ignore.

Perhaps the most articulate contemporary writer on this subject is the Australian ethicist Peter Singer, a philosopher in the utilitarian tradition who recently became Princeton University's first professor of bioethics. His faculty appointment, like his work in general, is exceedingly controversial because of his "radical" positions on a number of issues, including animal rights. In 1975, Singer published a best-selling book, *Animal Liberation,* that became the bible of the animal-rights movement (whose successes have included ending dog surgery in the training of medical students). Singer became a vegetarian while at Oxford University during the era of the Vietnam War, and he is most outspoken on the matter of humans' domination of other animals, which he considers a form of tyranny. I would refer you to his writings for a thoughtful, intelligent, and provocative discussion of the ethical problem arising from eating animals.

The ecological issue is less philosophical and more practical. Many meat eaters are simply not aware of the impact of their protein choices on the environment. Raising animals for meat wastes precious natural resources, including food and water, and it is a surprisingly important factor in the worsening pollution of soils, water tables, and air all over the planet. If Frances Moore Lappé was wrong about protein combining, she was right about the wastefulness of feeding nutritionally valuable grains to animals. Fed directly to people, those same grains would significantly reduce hunger and starvation worldwide. The inconceivable amounts of wastes produced by animals raised for meat create an impossible problem of disposal. Many of those wastes find their way into surface and groundwater, carrying with them residues of agrichemicals, drugs, and hormones. Even the flatulence of cows is troublesome: The methane expelled by cows the world over is now a significant factor in the depletion of the atmosphere's protective ozone layer. Some experts say that cows and cars do almost equal damage to the atmosphere and the environment in general.

The implications of relying on dairy products as protein sources are more complicated. As I noted above, the protein in milk is suspect as an allergen and irritant of the immune system in people with allergic family histories. In addition, milk provides the other two macronutrients in forms that can be problematic. Lactose, the sugar in milk, is the only carbohydrate of animal origin in our diets. Its digestion requires the enzyme lactase that many adults lack, causing them to suffer digestive distress if they drink milk or eat milk products containing lactose. People of northern European origin make lactase throughout life, but others, especially Asians and Africans, no longer produce it once they are weaned in infancy. For this reason, some nutritional experts strongly object to the dairy industry's intense promotion of milk as a necessary element of the diet, to meet calcium as well as protein needs. These critics consider the propaganda ethnocentric, if not racist, and advise that lactose-intolerant individuals and cultures look elsewhere for protein and calcium.

Moreover, butterfat, the fat in whole milk that becomes highly concentrated in cream, ice cream, cheese, and, of course, butter is the most saturated of the animal fats, delivering a whopping 54 percent of SFAs. Butterfat in the Western diet, particularly in the form of cheese, is probably the greatest single contributor to the overload of saturated fat responsible for the high rates of cardiovascular disease in our societies. Butterfat is also one of the only natural sources of *trans*-fatty acids, formed as a result of bacterial transformation of unsaturated fatty acids in the stomachs of cows. (They account for a relatively small percentage of dietary TFAs compared to margarine and partially hydrogenated vegetable oils.)

Cow's milk contains much more fat than human milk, and people love the mouth feel and flavor of butterfat. I and most people I know love cheese, even though we eat it in moderation. We love it for its unctuous texture and complex range of flavors that includes notes of earth, mushrooms, and, in riper varieties, distinctly animal tones that in other contexts might be disagreeable. And the combination of sweet, fat, and cold in ice cream is almost irresistible. It is likely that some of our attraction to these foods has to do with the experience of nursing as the ultimate source of comfort and security.

I include some dairy products in my diet. I like cheese and note that it is part of the Mediterranean diet, which I consider a strong example of a healthful diet. I do not drink milk or use cream, rarely eat ice cream, and have come to replace almost all the butter I used to eat with olive oil. At the end of this section I will give you specific suggestions for using dairy products wisely. But I do want you to be aware of the reasons for not making them your main source of protein.

Aside from the hazards of its natural constituents, milk today may adversely affect health for other reasons. Unpasteurized milk can transmit serious infectious diseases (tuberculosis, brucellosis). Homogenization of milk, designed to prevent the cream from separating, changes the size of butterfat particles in ways that may make them more likely to contribute to atherosclerosis. Environmental toxins can accumulate in milk, especially in its fatty fraction. And drugs and hormones given to dairy cows to increase milk production will also find their way into "nature's most perfect food."

This last danger has become a focal point of contention because of the recent advent of recombinant bovine somatotropin (rBST), also known as bovine growth hormone (BGH), a synthetic hormone used to make dairy cows produce significantly more milk. The manufacturer of this product has promoted it heavily and spent a fortune to convince government agencies and consumers that BST presents no hazards to cows or people, only great economic benefits to dairy farmers. Consumers remain suspicious, as do I. The problem is that use of BGH can increase rates of mastitis—inflammation of udders—requiring greater use of antibiotics. Residues of antibiotics in milk contribute significantly to the development of antibiotic-resistant bacteria in people.

The milk of goats and sheep is mainly used to make cheese, but goat's milk is sometimes recommended as a substitute for cow's milk for children who are allergic or otherwise intolerant to casein. Goat's milk is somewhat closer to human milk in composition, but the milk fat of all these species is highly saturated and best consumed in moderation.

I would now like to discuss the remaining animal sources of protein—fish and shellfish—and then look at the pros and cons of vegetable protein from beans, grains, and nuts.

Fish and, even more so, shellfish appear to be less like us than cows, pigs, and sheep, so that eating them makes the ethical dilemma of living at the expense of other life recede a bit. Earlier I extolled the virtues of certain fish as sources of omega-3 fatty acids, particularly of the longer-chain members of that family, EPA and DHA, that the body may have difficulty synthesizing from the precursor (LNA, linolenic acid) that occurs in seeds and nuts. Epidemiological evidence consistently shows that populations eating fish have better health and longevity than those that don't and suggests that the more fish people eat, the better. Of course, many commonly eaten species of fish, such as halibut, flounder, cod, and sole, are not fatty and do not provide omega-3s; nonetheless, their inclusion in the diet seems to be healthy. Why?

One possibility is that people who eat a lot of fish do not eat a lot of meat and so take in less saturated fat. Another is that fish might contain other protective factors yet to be discovered. For much of history, fish has had the reputation of being the "poor man's meat." Ironically, as tastes have changed in the developed world, as more people have learned about the health benefits of eating fish, and, especially, as populations of fish throughout the world have dwindled as a result of overharvesting, the price of fish has increased enormously, often making it more expensive than meat.

Besides depleting fishing grounds once considered inexhaustible, like the Grand Banks off Newfoundland, human activity has harmed fish in another way, decreasing its value as a more healthful source of animal protein. Pollution of the world's oceans, lakes, and rivers with a great variety of industrial and agricultural wastes has put toxins into the food chains of which fish are a part. For saltwater species, the larger the fish, the more carnivorous it is, and the more time it spends in coastal waters where contaminated effluents are greatest, the likelier it is to have dangerous amounts of environmental toxins in its flesh. For freshwater fish, contamination is so great a concern that I advise shunning it altogether, unless you know for sure that the water it came from was unpolluted (there is not much of that left on the planet) or the fish is farm raised.

Fish-farming has its own problems. It is becoming big business, especially for salmon, trout, sturgeon, catfish, and tilapia. Farmed fish live in unnaturally crowded pens and are susceptible to diseases as a result. Farmers routinely give them antibiotics. The diseases incubated in these populations can escape to infect wild populations, sharply decreasing their numbers. Furthermore, unless the feed given to farmed fish is thoughtfully designed, their nutritional value may be less than that of their wild counterparts. This is an issue particularly with salmon. Farmed salmon contain fewer omega-3 fatty acids than wild salmon, unless, just as is the case with chickens, they get supplements of algae rich in those vital nutrients. Given the booming market for farmed salmon, I keep waiting for some clever entrepreneur to bring to market an organically raised, drug-free product with an omega-3 content equal to or greater than that of wild salmon.

The term *shellfish* applies to two very different kinds of animals: crustaceans and mollusks. Crustaceans include crabs, crayfish, lobsters, and shrimp. Their flesh contains cholesterol but little fat and provides high-quality protein. I won't go into the ethical issues involved in dropping them live into boiling water (and did you know that lobsters mate for life?), but I will say that their feeding habits pose certain risks to health. Crustaceans are scavengers and bottom feeders; they live in places where toxic pollutants accumulate. These creatures can be farmed, and if farmers take care to provide them with clean water, their value as protein foods is much higher.

Mollusks, such as clams, oysters, mussels, and scallops, are distant from us biologically, although octopus and squid, which are also in this category, have quite complex nervous systems and behavior. The practice of eating raw shellfish is particularly risky because of possible viral and bacterial infection. Serious diseases like hepatitis and cholera can be acquired in this way, and other shellfish-borne infections that would not bother most of us can be life-threatening for those with compromised immune systems (patients on immunosuppressive drugs and persons with AIDS). The possibility of toxic contamination here is also great. I like to spend time on islands in the Strait of Georgia between mainland British Columbia and Vancouver Island, an area famous for rich oyster beds that were a major protein source for the Native Americans who once dominated the region.

Today numerous paper mills discharge noxious effluents into the ocean, not only interfering with the reproduction of oysters but making them questionable as food.

That completes a survey of the common animal sources of protein. Before I leave the subject, I should note some general pros and cons of these foods. Many of them provide vitamins and minerals that the body needs. Meat, for example, is an important source of iron that is superior to vegetable sources because it is more bioavailable—that is, the body can use it more efficiently than iron in plants or supplements. For many people, milk and milk products are good sources of calcium. As a group, these foods provide many of the vitamins in the B complex. They are, however, devoid of two categories of micronutrients I will write about in the following section: fiber and phytochemicals, and one of the great problems associated with diets high in animal protein is deficiency of these protective factors. That may be another reason why epidemiologists consistently find an inverse correlation between the percentage of animal foods in the diet and better health.

Plant protein occurs in small amounts in leaves and some tubers and in much larger amounts in seeds. The seeds of pod-bearing plants, or legumes, are particularly rich sources. These include peas, beans, and lentils. All of them contain carbohydrate as well, of the low-glycemic-index sort, and a few—soybeans especially—contain significant amounts of fat. In addition, they are high in fiber, some vitamins (like folic acid, an important member of the B complex), and protective phytochemicals. There are several disadvantages of legumes as protein sources as well. They may be toxic raw; most require long cooking to make them palatable and digestible, and many contain resistant carbohydrates that cause flatulence and other digestive problems. They may also carry residues of toxic agrichemicals, a possibility I will discuss in the following section when I write about conventional versus organic agriculture.

Of all the legumes, soybeans deserve the most attention. Not only are they very high in protein, they have a heart-healthy oil that includes some omega-3 fatty acids. Also, as I mentioned earlier, they contain isoflavones, phytochemicals with hormonal effects that may protect both men and women from common forms of cancer. I will also write about the possible benefits (and risks) of isoflavones in the next section.

For centuries, East Asians have relied on soybeans as a staple, consuming them in a great many ways. They boil fresh, green soybeans in the pod (*edamame*), enjoying them hot or cold as we would eat peanuts. They make a protein-rich milk from the beans that they drink as is, or turn into tofu. The "skin" that forms on the surface of soy milk can be dried and used as the basis for creating a variety of mock meat products. Indonesians inoculate cooked soybeans with a mold culture that binds them into mild-flavored, solid cakes of *tempeh,* a unique food that lends itself to many different cooking methods.

In both China and Japan, vegetarian cuisines that developed in Buddhist temples rely heavily on soy foods. The Chinese tradition, which also uses a lot of gluten or wheat protein, has produced an astonishing variety of "facsimile foods" designed to resemble in appearance, texture, and flavor classic preparations of meat, fish, and fowl. I have enjoyed this food in restaurants in Shanghai, Hong Kong, and a number of cities in the United States, where menus offer dozens of dishes, everything from Peking duck and sweet-and-sour pork to braised fish, all of them purely vegetarian and fashioned from soy and gluten, using all of the varied flavor principles of Chinese cooking.

In Japan, Buddhist temple cuisine is called *shojin ryori* and is available at both temple restaurants and specialty restaurants not affiliated with Buddhist institutions. It is less concerned with fashioning imitations of animal foods and more focused on creating exquisite meals, as beautiful as those of the *kaiseki* cuisine that evolved as part of the formal tea ceremony. I remember a wonderful *shojin ryori* lunch I enjoyed with a friend at Nanzenji, a famous old Zen temple in Kyoto, on a sunny autumn day looking out over the temple gardens. The soy foods in it were ingenious and delicious.

Western food technology has also had a good run with soy. It has isolated soy protein from other components of the beans and fashioned it into all sorts of processed foods, from powdered protein drinks to nondairy frozen desserts and vegetarian hot dogs, pepperoni, and cheese. In fact, the amazing versatility of soy has resulted in such a profusion of products that people wishing to add soybeans to their diets may be totally confused.

I think you would do well to learn about soy foods and eat more of them. Substituting them for some of the animal foods in the standard Western diet would be a healthful change, perhaps one of the most healthful changes you could make. At one stroke, you would decrease intake of saturated fat and increase omega-3s, fiber, and protective phytochemicals. You would also eat lower on the food chain and so lessen your exposure to environmental toxins, not to mention the drugs and hormones in meat.

Some soy products taste terrible. If you have been turned off by them, keep experimenting, because there are now some quite delicious soy foods on the market. Be aware that highly processed soy foods (those made with "isolated soy protein") may not contain the isoflavones, fiber, and healthful oil of the whole bean. Again, read labels carefully. I recommend that you also try to get products made from organically grown soybeans, since pesticides are used heavily on this crop.

One of the best soy foods to start with is *edamame,* which is delicious and fun to eat. All you have to do is boil the whole green beans in salted water until they are tender (about ten minutes). Japanese eat them cold as a summer snack with beer, and sushi bars offer them as an appetizer, either warm or cold. You pop the beans out of their pods directly into your mouth (and discard the pods). I am happy to report that since I first wrote about *edamame* three years ago, they have become much more widely available. Look for them fresh or frozen (or even precooked) at specialty produce stores, Asian groceries, and even some supermarkets.

Many people I know like roasted "soy nuts," small, whole beans that have been dry-roasted or roasted in oil and seasoned. Read labels of these products to make sure they have not been cooked in an unhealthful oil. I am much less enthusiastic about "soy butter," an alternative to peanut butter; the brands I have tried all have a funny, beany taste.

Many brands of soy milk on the market are good. You have a wide choice of products, from full fat to nonfat, plain, sweetened, or flavored, and calcium fortified. Some taste better than others. You can substitute soy milk for cow's milk in most recipes and give it to children who have been advised not to drink cow's milk. People who want to avoid dairy products may like soy cheeses; most of them contain some casein (milk protein) to make the texture and melting qualities more like those of regular cheese. Some precooked soy burgers on the market are remarkably meatlike, as are some soy sausages, hot dogs, and lunch meats. They are much more healthful, especially for kids, than standard versions made from meat. Find brands you like, and check labels to make sure the ingredients are acceptable.

If you find that soy upsets your digestion and gives you gas, you should avoid certain products altogether. Soy grits, soy flour, and texturized vegetable protein (TVP) are the worst offenders. *Edamame* and *tempeh* should not bother you. If you are allergic to soy or very sensitive to digestive upsets from it, you may be able to tolerate it if you introduce it very slowly. Try eating a tiny amount of soy—a few *edamame,* a swallow of soy milk, or a bite of tofu—every day for a couple of weeks, then very slowly increase the amount. There is a good chance of building tolerance to this valuable protein source in this way.

I do not mean to slight other legumes by devoting so many words to soy. Many beans contain isoflavones and other protective micronutrients, including fiber and folic acid, along with quality protein and carbohydrate. Beans are filling and satisfying, especially when they are cooked to sufficient tenderness and artfully flavored. Lentils, a mainstay of Indian cuisine, cook quickly and can be turned into tasty purées and soups. I buy jars of spicy, nonfat, black-bean dips that I serve as snacks to be eaten with carrot sticks or chips, and I often make *hummus,* the Middle Eastern appetizer made from puréed chickpeas (garbanzos) and sesame and flavored with fresh lemon juice, olive oil, and garlic. If you experience flatulence from beans, avoid those varieties with the highest content of resistant carbohydrate (pink beans, for example) and use those with the lowest (like black beans, Anasazi beans, and chickpeas).

Grains provide protein along with carbohydrate, but only wheat protein lends itself to the sort of alchemy that can be done with soy. Gluten "develops" when wheat flour and water are kneaded; it is what gives a stretchy, springy quality to dough as well as body and character to good bread. If you knead a ball of dough in water, you can actually separate the gluten from the starch that accompanies it. I used to do this at home, repeatedly pouring off the milky, starch-filled water and replacing it with fresh water, until it remained clear. By that time, the dough would be one-third of its original size and look like a mass of rubber bands—mostly gluten. You can simmer this homemade gluten in a broth or cut it in pieces and fry it, then use it as a replacement for animal protein. You can also buy canned, flavored gluten in Chinese grocery stores under such names as "mock duck" and "mock abalone," and add it to stir-fried vegetables, for a quick, delicious main dish.

Since the invention of agriculture, grain-based diets have certainly prevented protein deficiency in many parts of the world. As long as the grains are not highly processed to eliminate their fiber and other micronutrients and raise the glycemic index of their starch content, foods prepared from them are healthful.

Some seeds (sesame, sunflower) and nuts (almonds, walnuts, hazelnuts) are rich in protein, but they contain too much fat to be useful as primary protein sources. I have already recommended including some nuts in the diet—say, a small handful a day—for their good oils, as well as fiber and other micronutrients (vitamin E, trace minerals). The protein they provide is an extra benefit. I often make nut milk, mostly from blanched, raw almonds or raw cashews, and use it as a healthful substitute for dairy cream in some recipes. The procedure is simple. Grind a half cup of nuts in a blender until very fine, then add one to two cups of cold water and blend the mixture on high speed for two minutes. The amount of water you add will determine the richness of the nut milk, which you can sweeten or flavor (with vanilla extract, for example).

Getting your protein from vegetable rather than animal foods has a number of advantages. Vegetable protein foods are cheaper and less perishable than meat and other flesh foods. Being lower on the food chain, they are less likely to have high concentrations of environmental toxins. The fat that accompanies their protein is better for you than animal fat, being much lower in SFAs. Vegetable protein also contains fiber and other micronutrients that animal foods lack. Because it contains fiber and carbohydrate, it is less concentrated than animal protein, so you can eat a greater volume of it without overloading your system with protein.

Finally, I should mention two other sources of dietary protein: mushrooms and powdered supplements meant to be blended into high-protein drinks and shakes.

Mushrooms are neither vegetables nor plants, being properly classified in a separate biological kingdom more closely related to animals. We actually share more DNA sequences with mushrooms than we do with plants, and to me their flesh, when well-cooked, resembles animal tissue more than plant tissue. You may have heard that mushrooms have little nutritional value. That is not so; they have a respectable content of protein along with trace minerals and vitamins. Unless you forage for wild mushrooms, one of my favorite hobbies, you probably eat just one species of edible mushroom, the common white or brown button mushroom or its large, mature form, the portobello. Increasingly, popular Asian mushrooms are appearing in Western markets and restaurants: shiitake, oyster mushrooms, enokidake, and maitake. And wild species, like morels, chanterelles, and porcini, are more available as well. I recommend getting to know them. In addition to their interesting flavors and textures, many of these offer important health benefits, such as reduction of serum cholesterol, enhancement of immunity, and some protection from cancer. But do not eat mushrooms raw—they contain toxins that cooking destroys.

The protein powders that fill the shelves of health food shops and drugstores are mainly used by young bodybuilders, obsessed with body image and "bulking up." The protein in them comes from soy or whey, the watery fraction of cow's milk left over after removal of the curds, which contain most of the protein and fat. Whey still has considerable protein and can be dried and powdered as a dietary supplement. Some people swear by it, and manufacturers make all sorts of health claims for it. I have no objection to the use of these supplements by people whose diets are deficient for one reason or another, such as those recovering from illness or old people unable to get nutritionally adequate meals. I think it is unwise to add them to a diet already rich in protein because of the danger of stressing the liver and kidneys. If you do use the powders, read the lists of ingredients carefully to make sure they do not include partially hydrogenated oils or unhealthful additives.

To sum up all of the recommendations about protein in the diet:

- Try to maintain protein intake between 10 and 20 percent of total calories. If you have liver or kidney problems, keep to the low end of this range or lower.
- If you have allergic problems or an autoimmune disease, try cutting down on protein to see if symptoms improve after one or two months. Avoid milk protein and reduce consumption of all animal protein.

- Try to substitute vegetable protein, especially soy foods, for some of the animal protein in your diet.
- Reduce consumption of beef or substitute bison, drug- and hormone-free beef from free-range cattle, or wild game.
- If you eat chicken, get drug- and hormone-free, free-range chicken, and remove some or all of the skin and fat before cooking.
- If you eat eggs, use omega-3 fortified, organically raised eggs from free-range chickens.
- Minimize consumption of cured meats (including bacon, salami, lunch meats, and hot dogs) made with nitrates and nitrites, which can form carcinogens in the stomach. Try to substitute products made from turkey or use vegetarian versions made from soy and wheat gluten.
- Never eat brains. Minimize consumption of other organ meats.
- If you or your spouse is allergic, do not give your children cow's milk or milk products until they are two or, better, three years old. Use soy milk and other soy products instead.
- Read labels of dairy products you use to learn their fat content and figure it into your total saturated fat consumption. If you like cheese, use natural varieties made with part-skim milk and strong-flavored varieties like Parmesan that can be used in moderate quantities to season dishes. Try to stay away from cheeses with total fat content greater than 70 percent of calories.
- Try to eat more fish and to eat it in place of other animal foods. Of the fish rich in omega-3s, the best are sardines (packed in water) and wild Alaskan salmon. Smoked salmon is fine if it does not contain unhealthful additives. Make a real effort not to eat swordfish, marlin, shark, or other very large, carnivorous fish; they are likely to contain unhealthful levels of environmental toxins. The best ways to cook fish are broiling, grilling, steaming, and poaching as opposed to frying, pan-roasting, or baking with a lot of butter. Raw fish served in good Japanese restaurants and sushi bars is fine.
- Minimize consumption of shellfish unless you know it comes from clean waters. Be very careful about eating raw mollusks. Try not to decrease the nutritional benefits of these protein foods by cooking them in unhealthful amounts of saturated fat (or drowning them in melted butter at the table).
- Incorporate soy foods into your diet. Familiarize yourself with the

great variety of soy products in natural food stores and regular supermarkets to find those you like, and favor those made from organically grown soybeans. Read labels of processed soy foods carefully to check for fat content (below 30 percent of calories is desirable) and the presence of unhealthful ingredients and additives. If soy causes allergic symptoms or indigestion, try introducing it in very small amounts every day and increase intake gradually.

- Eat beans and other legumes frequently as protein sources. If they cause you digestive problems, experiment with different varieties to find ones that agree with you.
- Eat a variety of whole grains, preferably in less refined, less processed forms.
- Eat moderate quantities of protein- (and oil-) rich nuts and seeds.
- Learn to cook and enjoy the different types of mushrooms now available. Never eat any mushrooms raw, and always cook them thoroughly to improve their digestibility and nutritional value.
- Avoid protein powders as supplements to diets already providing adequate protein. If you use protein powders instead of protein foods, read the labels carefully to select those that are free of unhealthful ingredients and additives (such as saturated fat, partially hydrogenated oils, or artificial colors).

Those are the best suggestions I can give you about the third and last macronutrient. It is now time to look at the micronutrients.

V

THE MICRONUTRIENTS

Your body needs micronutrients in much smaller amounts than macronutrients—a few millionths of a gram a day in the case of some vitamins and minerals—but that does not mean they are of less importance than sources of caloric energy and structural materials. Deficiencies of some of these dietary elements will result in certain sickness and death, and of others in impairment of the body's defenses and suboptimal functioning of many of its systems. The four classes of micronutrients you need to know about are vitamins, minerals, fiber, and protective phytochemicals.

VITAMINS

Vitamins were an early-twentieth-century discovery and are now a bonanza for manufacturers and merchants of dietary supplements. A diverse group of compounds, vitamins are essential nutrients obtainable from a normal diet that are necessary for health and growth. Some occur mainly in plants (vitamins C and E, for example), some mainly in animal tissue (the B complex), and some in both. The body can make vitamin D from a form of cholesterol on exposure to the ultraviolet radiation in sunlight, and bacteria in the gut make limited amounts of B vitamins and vitamin K. Eating a widely varied diet provides the best insurance against vitamin deficiency; the more restrictive the diet, the higher the chances of not getting what you need.

Vitamin-deficiency diseases are rare in our societies today, in part because these micronutrients are added to many foods. For instance, white flour and breakfast cereals are enriched with the B-complex group that is removed from whole grains during milling, and milk is often "fortified" with synthetic vitamin D. Furthermore, increasing numbers of people are taking vitamins every day in the form of supplements. Is it necessary to take supplements if you are eating a varied and balanced diet? I will give you my opinion on that as I explain the different vitamins.

Vitamins fall into two groups: those that are water-soluble (B complex and C) and those that are fat-soluble (A, D, E, and K).

The water-soluble vitamins are widely distributed in actively metabolizing tissues, suggesting their importance in regulating the enzyme-mediated reactions by which the body obtains energy from carbohydrates, fats, and proteins. The B vitamins, in particular, function as coenzymes, binding to enzymes and allowing them to function as metabolic catalysts. Vitamin C is primarily a chemical reducing agent that regulates metabolic reactions and forms a keystone of the body's defense system against oxidative stress. It is also needed for the synthesis of connective tissue and maintenance of normal vascular structure and function.

We used to think that the water-soluble vitamins were completely nontoxic, even in megadoses, because it is so easy for the body to eliminate excess amounts in urine, but we now know that too much C can disturb gastrointestinal and urinary function and that several of the B vitamins can be harmful if used in too-large quantities. Vitamin B₃—niacin—which is prescribed in high dosage to lower serum cholesterol, can cause derangement of liver function, including a devastating form of toxic hepatitis. Too much vitamin B₆—pyridoxine—can damage peripheral nerves, causing progressive numbness that patients and doctors can mistake for a symptom of multiple sclerosis.

Therefore it is important to get the right amounts of vitamins, because either too much or too little can be problematic. The recommended daily allowances (RDAs) set by government agencies were determined only with a view to preventing deficiency states, not to promoting optimum health or treating specific medical conditions. The amount of vitamin C that provides the maximum defense against oxidative stress is higher than the amount that prevents scurvy. The amount of niacin that treats stubborn hypercholesterolemia is much greater than the amount that prevents pellagra. If you are a smoker or a habitual drinker, your vitamin needs may be increased. Alcohol destroys vitamin B₁—thiamine—for example, and unless regular drinkers take supplemental thiamine, they are at greater risk for the development of central nervous system problems associated with alcoholism.

Finding the optimal dosage for vitamin C has been a focus of intense controversy. The late Linus Pauling advocated megadosing, up to eighteen grams (18,000 milligrams) a day, three hundred times the RDA of 60 milligrams. But recent research, including a study conducted by Balz Frei, Ph.D., director of the Linus Pauling Institute, makes clear that the body simply cannot use these amounts; its tissues become saturated with the vitamin at doses of 120 to 200 milligrams. Any excess spills over into the urine, and high doses routinely cause flatulence, loose stools, diarrhea, and, in some individuals, urinary frequency and urgency. It is also clear that 60 milligrams is too little to provide optimum antioxidant benefits.

Vitamin C occurs naturally in ripe fruits and some vegetables (notably red peppers). Most animals synthesize the vitamin C they need from moment to moment, but humans and other primates have lost this ability, and since we also cannot store vitamin C, we need to take it in regularly. If your diet includes a lot of fresh fruits and vegetables, you may not need to take any supplementally, but you still might want to for insurance; if your diet does not include a lot of these foods, supplementing would definitely be a good idea. I take about 100 milligrams twice a day.

I also take a B-complex supplement every day, mainly to be sure I'm getting enough folic acid, one of the unnumbered B vitamins. Folic acid, found in green leafy vegetables (the name comes from *foliage*) as well as beans and orange juice, is deficient in the diets of many Westerners. It is important, along with vitamins B6 and B12, in regulating levels of homocysteine, a toxic amino acid formed in the metabolic breakdown of protein, especially animal protein. A high level of homocysteine in the blood is an independent risk factor for arterial disease and heart attack and may also elevate the risk of cancer and a number of chronic degenerative diseases. The body can easily clear homocysteine from the blood if it has adequate amounts of vitamins B6, B12, and, especially, folic acid. You should be taking in about 800 micrograms of folic acid a day; if you get 400 micrograms from a B-complex supplement, the rest will come from a normal diet. If your diet includes a lot of animal protein and not a lot of fresh fruits and vegetables, it is especially important to supplement it with folic acid. (Any woman contemplating pregnancy should not fail to do this. Folic acid deficiency in the earliest stages of pregnancy, before the condition announces itself, may cause spina bifida and other neural tube defects—devastating fetal abnormalities.)

Vitamin B12 deserves comment as the sole member of this group found only in foods of animal origin. People who follow vegan diets (those that include no eggs, dairy products, or other animal foods) are at risk for B12 deficiency, which results in a distinctive form of anemia and nerve damage. The body can store this vitamin and needs only minuscule amounts of it each day, so that even if dietary supplies are cut off, symptoms of deficiency may not appear for a very long time. Growing children on vegan diets are more at risk; they will get sick and not develop properly unless they get B12 in supplement form. This is part of the reason I think that the optimum diet should not be vegan but should include some fish, eggs, or dairy products.

The fat-soluble vitamins are more diverse and probably less well understood than the water-soluble group. Excess intake of two of them, vitamins A and D, can cause serious toxicity, but cases of that are extremely rare and mostly concern people taking unusual amounts of vitamin supplements. No known toxicity is associated with vitamins E and K.

Vitamin D mostly regulates absorption and utilization of calcium (and phosphorus) and the mineralization of bone. The major source of it is synthesis within the body as a result of ultraviolet irradiation of the skin—i.e., sun exposure. Although it occurs naturally in fish-liver oils, butter, and egg yolk, the main dietary source is now fortified milk.

Deficiency of vitamin D can be an important contributing factor to osteoporosis, the demineralization of bones that affects the elderly, and is more likely to occur in people living at northern latitudes in the winter and those who are shut in. As a longtime resident of southern Arizona, I have been unconcerned about the need for vitamin D in the diet, but recent research convinces me that deficiency of this micronutrient is more common than I thought, even in people living in the Sun Belt. It may not be a bad idea for everyone to take 400 IU (international units) a day in supplement form, making up the rest of the body's requirement from time in the sun. Women are at risk of osteoporosis (due to declining levels of sex hormones) much earlier in life than men; they should seek out calcium supplements that include this amount of vitamin D. By the way, the amount of time in the sun the body requires for vitamin D synthesis is quite small, perhaps as little as fifteen minutes a day, but be aware that sunscreens block the reaction.

The body needs vitamin K for normal coagulation of the blood. It gets it from intestinal synthesis by normal gut flora as well as from the diet, primarily from vegetables such as broccoli and leafy greens. Deficiency of vitamin K, resulting in abnormal bleeding, is quite rare, occurring mainly in patients who are very sick (with advanced liver disease, for example) or who are unable to absorb the vitamin from the intestinal tract. (Affluence and improved sanitation have ironically raised the risk of acute vitamin K deficiency in newborn babies, who today might not have the rich gut flora they need to synthesize it and that babies in less hygienic environments have. That is the reason doctors give newborns a prophylactic injection of vitamin K.)

Doctors routinely suppress synthesis of vitamin K in patients at risk for blood clots by giving them anticoagulant drugs like warfarin (Coumadin), commonly known as blood thinners. Patients on anticoagulant therapy can undo the protection they get from it by eating too many vitamin-K-rich vegetables (or consuming too much green tea, which contains an especially high concentration of vitamin K).

The actions of vitamin A are more complex. It is necessary for normal vision and function of the retina, maintains the health of skin and tissues that cover surfaces of organs, and participates in some metabolic reactions. The vitamin itself occurs in such animal foods as fish-liver oils, liver, egg yolk, butter, and cream, but beta carotene (also known as provitamin A), which the body can use to make it, is widely distributed in yellow and orange fruits and vegetables and dark, leafy greens. Unlike vitamin A, which can accumulate in tissues and cause toxicity in high doses, beta carotene is water-soluble and nontoxic, although people who eat a lot of it, either in natural sources or supplements, may turn orange, a harmless and reversible, if striking, change in appearance.

Beta-carotene-rich fruits and vegetables also contain a number of other, related pigments, collectively known as carotenoids. (Some of the others are alpha carotene, cryptoxanthin, zeaxanthin, lutein, and lycopene, the last being the red pigment in tomatoes, pink grapefruit, and watermelon.) This important group of phytochemicals, which I will have more to say about, is now being studied intensely for its cancer-preventive properties, and researchers are also working with various vitamin-A derivatives as new cancer treatments that are less toxic than conventional forms of chemotherapy.

Most people on normal diets will get enough preformed vitamin A or enough of the provitamin to make what their bodies need. I think there is good reason, however, to think about increasing intake of the carotenoid pigments because of their antioxidant properties and their ability to reduce cancer risks. The best way to do this is to increase consumption of fruits and vegetables that contain them. If you take them in the form of a supplement, it is important to get as many members of the family as you can in one capsule.

Finally, vitamin E, long ignored by physicians and dieticians, is now recognized as another cornerstone of the body's defense system against oxidative stress. It has the special function of preventing oxidation of the polyunsaturated fatty acids in membranes and cells (thereby reducing cancer risks), and probably is necessary for normal nerve and muscle function. We have a lot more to learn about it.

Dietary sources of vitamin E are oil-rich seeds and nuts and the oils expressed from them, the embryo (germ) of whole grains, especially wheat, leafy vegetables, legumes, and egg yolks. Disease due to deficiency of vitamin E is rare, but many people might not be getting enough of it to enjoy optimum health and protection from degenerative disease. High doses of vitamin E have useful therapeutic effects. Applied topically to closed wounds, they reduce scar formation; taken internally, they reduce symptoms of fibrocystic breasts, alleviate menstrual and premenstrual problems, and act as a natural blood thinner, reducing risk of heart attack.

Vitamin E is actually a group of related compounds called tocopherols; alpha, beta, gamma, and delta tocopherols occur together in foods, but because alpha-tocopherol is the most active, most medical research has focused on it, and most vitamin E supplements provide it alone. Because tocopherols are asymmetric molecules, they can exist in mirror-image forms. The right-hand forms are the *d*-isomers, and the left-hand forms are the *l*-isomers. Only the right-hand forms are active, but synthetic vitamin E, the usual kind in supplements, is an equal mixture of both. So this is the one case where a meaningful distinction exists between the natural and synthetic forms of a vitamin. For the other vitamins, buying more expensive natural forms is a waste of money, no matter what the manufacturers claim. But with vitamin E it is most important to buy a natural product—*d*-alpha tocopherol plus the other members of the family: beta-, gamma-, and delta-tocopherols. A recent study suggests that gamma-tocopherol is more powerful than alpha-tocopherol in preventing cancer. There is none of it in synthetic vitamin E.

The government has set the RDA for vitamin E extremely low: 30 IU. Most experts on nutritional medicine agree that daily doses of 400 to 800 IU are necessary for maximum antioxidant effect, optimum health, and surest disease prevention. It is not possible to get these amounts from food; you would have to eat more than a pound of nuts to do so, giving you far too many fat calories. I recommend taking natural vitamin E as a dietary supplement. Take it with a meal that includes fat to ensure its absorption.

The best way to guarantee that you get all the vitamins you need is to eat a varied diet containing plenty of fresh fruits and vegetables, whole grains, and nuts and seeds as well as some of the more healthful animal foods, and to spend some time in the sun. In addition, I suggest taking a B-complex supplement that provides 400 micrograms of folic acid, additional vitamin C—say, 100 milligrams twice a day—a capsule of mixed carotenoids, and 400 to 800 IU of natural vitamin E. Those at risk for osteoporosis should also consider taking 400 IU of supplemental vitamin D.

MINERALS

Prior to 1930, doctors and nutritionists paid little attention to most of the minerals now known to be essential for life and health. They knew that iron was necessary to make red blood cells and iodine was needed to prevent goiter, but they had no idea of the human body's need for copper, zinc, selenium, or other "trace minerals." I won't discuss the particular requirements for, and functions of, each of the twenty-eight naturally occurring essential elements. Rather, I will write about those that seem to me to be especially important in designing the optimum diet. I will also save you a great deal of time and trouble by condensing my advice about minerals to a very few words: eat more fruits and vegetables.

Walk into a health food store (or drugstore, for that matter) and you will see a great many single-mineral and multimineral supplements for sale, sometimes combined with vitamins. Two years ago, I was receiving promotional audiotapes and literature for a liquid multimineral supplement that was very expensive. The company's expert spokesman, a veterinarian, claimed that most human diseases were due to unrecognized mineral deficiencies and were curable by taking regular doses of the product. He added that fruits and vegetables were no longer trustworthy sources of these micronutrients because of modern growing methods and depleted soils. This is all nonsense.

In general, I see no need to take any multimineral products unless you are on a severely restricted diet. People whose diets are deficient in particular minerals can certainly benefit from supplementation, but this must be determined on a case-by-case basis. For example, iodine deficiency (and prevalence of goiter) is not uncommon in populations living far from the sea who do not eat seafood or sea vegetables. Iodized salt has been a blessing for them. Many persons with adult-onset diabetes are deficient in chromium and will have better blood sugar levels if they take that mineral in supplemental form. But taking more of those minerals if you do not need them is not going to improve health and may have harmful effects. There is no evidence, for example, to support the claims of supplement manufacturers that chromium pills improve carbohydrate metabolism and promote weight loss in normal people.

The minerals that require a bit of discussion because of their importance to general health are iron, calcium, sodium, potassium, selenium, and zinc.

Iron-deficiency anemia—when the body makes fewer and smaller red blood cells, with consequent reduced capacity to transport and use oxygen—used to be a very common diagnosis. Fifty years ago, doctors, nurses, pharmacists, and dietitians were quick to give this label to anyone complaining of fatigue or lack of energy and to recommend iron tonics as the cure. Today, simple blood tests are used to diagnose iron-deficiency anemia, for which the commonest cause is blood loss of some sort that must be identified, and we know that supplemental iron can be dangerously toxic if you don't need it. The body cannot eliminate iron except through blood loss. Other than women who menstruate heavily, healthy people should not take iron supplements. Iron is an oxidizing agent—the sort of thing antioxidants protect us from—and too much of it in the body can promote unhealthy changes in cells, increasing risks of cardiovascular disease and cancer. Some people with abnormal liver function can develop iron overload disease, a life-threatening condition, if they take in too much of this element.

So never take supplemental iron unless a blood test shows you to have iron-deficiency anemia (and if you do have it, make sure you and your doctor work together to find the cause) or you are pregnant, nursing, or have lost a lot of blood. If you are not in those categories, read labels of any multivitamin products you use to make sure they do not contain iron. Children, however, do have increased iron needs, and pediatricians can advise you how best to provide for them.

Meat eaters get plenty of iron from the skeletal muscles of animals, and it is in an easily assimilable form. Vegetarians may not get plenty of iron and may have a harder time absorbing and using what they do eat. They tend to have slightly lower iron and hemoglobin levels than meat eaters, but some experts think that this difference, far from being a disadvantage, may correlate with lower risk of cardiovascular disease (as a result of lower exposure to the pro-oxidant effects of iron). Because I recommend that you try to decrease consumption of meat, it is important for you to know the other sources of iron. Iron occurs in dried beans, some dried fruit (prunes, raisins, figs), molasses, green vegetables (especially dark, leafy greens), and cocoa. You can also get it by doing some of your cooking in (uncoated) iron pots. Vitamin C promotes the absorption of iron, so if you need more of it, try taking 100 milligrams of C along with meals containing iron-rich foods.

We hear a great deal about calcium these days because bones deficient in it are weak and susceptible to injury. Hip fractures in older people, often with osteoporosis as the underlying cause, are a common cause of disability and death. Because calcium is critical to nerve, muscle, cardiovascular, and kidney function, the body regulates blood levels of it very carefully, taking account of dietary intake and urinary loss, and drawing on the huge reservoir of this element in the bones. Many factors affect this equation, including hormones from the parathyroid and sex glands, exercise or lack of it, and other aspects of diet. For example, I wrote earlier that high-protein diets, particularly those high in dense animal protein, increase calcium loss in the urine. Wheat bran, raw spinach, fructose (as in high-fructose corn syrup in soft drinks), salt, caffeine, alcohol, and tobacco can all interfere with calcium absorption.

The dairy industry engages in heavy-handed promotion of milk and milk products as ideal sources of calcium. Sources of calcium they are, but as I have said, that comes together with lactose, casein, and butterfat, which are not so good for many of us. I eat modest amounts of dairy products, mostly cheese, but I make an effort to get calcium elsewhere as well. If you like sardines, those with bones are one good source; you will not notice the bones when you mash them up and season them as you like. Leafy greens such as collards and kale are also good, as are broccoli and the various sea vegetables (dulse, nori, and kombu, for example). Sesame seeds and sesame tahini are high in calcium, and yet another source is tofu, if the manufacturer used calcium chloride to coagulate the soy milk used to make it. Read the labels of tofu packages to see if this element is in the list of ingredients.

A number of foods on the market are now fortified with calcium, among them orange juice and soy milk. These are especially good for kids. If you use soy milk, yogurt, or cheese as substitutes for cow's milk products, be sure to buy calcium-fortified brands. Nutritionists recommend a daily calcium intake of 1,200 to 1,500 milligrams. If you are not eating calcium-rich foods regularly, you would do well to take this mineral in supplement form. Since supplemental calcium is harmless (and even has some beneficial relaxant effects on muscles and nerves), I think all persons at risk for osteoporosis and all whose diets are not high in calcium-rich foods—men as well as women—should take supplemental calcium.

Sodium, even more critical to normal body function than calcium, is under very tight control, since even slight deviations from normal blood levels have catastrophic results. We mostly take in sodium as sodium chloride—table salt—and eliminate it in sweat and urine. The only healthy people who have to worry about sodium deficiency are those who exercise vigorously in hot environments and don't replenish the salt lost through perspiration. They can become weak, faint, and disoriented as a result of excessive sodium loss. The rest of us would do better to worry about sodium excess.

Liking salt is a learned taste that some would call an addiction. Cows, deer, and other herbivores crave salt and travel long distances to find it; carnivores get the sodium they need from the blood and tissues of the animals they eat. Human craving for salt may date back only to the beginning of agriculture. Surviving hunter-gatherers who live mainly on wild game—some Amazonian Indians, for instance—neither know salt nor seek it out. Once humans came to like salt, they valued it highly; it has been a precious commodity throughout much of history.

Today, however, many medical experts identify salt as a primary cause of high blood pressure and all the problems associated with it, including increased risks of stroke, heart failure, and kidney failure. The evidence here is contradictory. It is clear that people with these problems do better on sodium-restricted diets, but whether eating excessive salt caused the problems is not clear.

Significant fractions of the population are salt-sensitive to one degree or another. Too much dietary salt can cause them to retain fluid, increasing circulatory volume and thereby adding to the workload of the heart and kidneys. Fluid retention can result in headaches and noticeable swelling of the hands and other parts of the body, especially in women. People who are not salt-sensitive may be able to handle any amount of dietary sodium without difficulty.

The foods in our diets that are very high in sodium are mostly processed foods, which are unhealthful in other ways. (Salt acts as a natural preservative as well as a flavor enhancer.) Eliminating or cutting way down on processed foods is one of the best ways to reduce your sodium intake and improve your diet. You can also train yourself to like lower levels of salt in food: by not adding salt at the table, by not eating snack foods (pretzels, chips, nuts) coated in salt, and by rinsing or soaking high-sodium foods like pickles, olives, and sauerkraut in fresh water to reduce their saltiness. Another strategy is to increase your intake of potassium, because these two elements work together in complementary ways.

Potassium abounds in fruits and vegetables. Almost all fruits are rich sources, as are starchy roots and dark, leafy greens. The ratio of sodium to potassium in the diet and in the system may be more determinative of long-range heart and kidney health than the level of sodium alone, and it is not hard to see why the ordinary diet, high in animal and processed foods and low in fruits and vegetables, would provide an unhealthful sodium/potassium ratio. The best solution is simply to increase intake of the latter, in other words, to *eat more fruits and vegetables*. You should never take supplemental potassium except on the orders of a physician, but you should definitely find ways to increase consumption of the natural sources of this element.

Selenium is truly a trace mineral, needed in microgram amounts to participate in the body's antioxidant defense system. It works in tandem with vitamin E to protect unsaturated fatty acids in membranes and cells from oxidation. Selenium occurs in protein-rich plant foods like seeds and nuts, but the amounts present depend on the levels of selenium in the soil in which the crops grew. Areas of the world with low soil selenium and consequent low levels in foods have higher cancer rates than those with high soil selenium, and contemporary research has documented powerful cancer-protective effects of this mineral. Brazil nuts are a good source, since two a day provide what the body needs. I take 200 micrograms a day of supplemental selenium with my vitamin E, and I recommend that to everyone as part of an antioxidant formula that also includes a capsule of mixed carotenoids (providing 25,000 IU of beta carotene along with alpha carotene, lutein, lycopene, and zeaxanthin), and the dose of vitamin C indicated above. Selenium can be toxic in amounts above 1,000 micrograms a day; the early signs of toxicity are peeling of fingernails and brittleness of hair.

As for zinc, vegetarians get less of this trace mineral than omnivores, and zinc from nonmeat sources is less available to the body. Vegetables and fruits provide little, but legumes (including soy products), nuts, eggs, and whole grains contain it, and wheat germ is an especially good source. Although deficiency of zinc can compromise immunity and many other functions of the body, you should be able to get enough of it without taking a supplement, even if you eat few animal foods, by making sure that you eat foods from the list above.

One last point: I meet people who object to drinking distilled and purified water because it has been "robbed" of its mineral content. We get trace minerals from foods, especially fruits and vegetables, not from water, and the benefits of purifying drinking water are myriad. It is your best protection against ingesting a host of toxins and pollutants that are serious threats to health.

FIBER

Fiber, otherwise known as roughage, is the indigestible part of food that makes up much of the bulk of stool. Though not a source of calories, vitamins, or minerals, it contributes to health in several ways, and deficiency of it in the ordinary diet is a significant nutritional problem in our societies. There are a number of different types of fiber, all of them "resistant carbohydrates," too complex for our digestive systems to break down. Vegetarians take in a lot of fiber. People who eat mainly meat, potatoes, and white bread do not. Although hard scientific evidence is lacking to support some of the claims made by fiber enthusiasts, I think most of us can benefit by eating more of it.

Fiber falls into two groups with respect to solubility in water. Insoluble fiber includes cellulose and lignin, which occur in whole grains, especially in wheat bran, and hemicellulose, which is slightly soluble in water and occurs in whole grains, nuts, seeds, fruits, and vegetables. Collectively, these insoluble fibers protect the health of the intestinal tract by increasing stool bulk and decreasing its transit time. They protect against such common conditions as irritable bowel syndrome and diverticulitis. Psyllium seed, widely cultivated in India, is a good source of hemicellulose and the main ingredient in "bulk laxatives" that make stools larger, softer, and easier to pass.

Gums and pectins are the two kinds of water-soluble fiber. The former occur in some grains and seeds—oats and sesame, for example—as well as in some legumes and trees that are sources of gums used in manufactured foods to improve their texture (for example, gum arabic, gum tragacanth, and gum karaya). Pectins are present in fruits, vegetables, and seeds, and purified fruit pectin is available for use as a jelling agent for homemade jams. Soluble fiber binds bile acids and cholesterol in the intestinal tract, preventing their reabsorption. For this reason, increasing soluble fiber in the diet can help lower serum cholesterol—a major selling point for oat bran in recent years.

I would try to eat 40 grams of fiber a day, about twice what most people get. The easiest way to do this is simply to eat more fruits and vegetables. Raspberries are one of the richest sources (one cup contains 40 grams); their fiber is in the tiny seeds. Cooked beans give you 4 grams of fiber in each half-cup serving. You should also try to eat more whole grains and products made from them, including cereals containing bran. To be worthwhile as a fiber source, a cereal should give you at least 4 and preferably 5 grams of bran per one-ounce serving.

Because fiber is a resistant carbohydrate, eating more of it may cause flatulence and bloating for the same reason that beans are gas producing. Bacteria in the gut attack and digest the complex carbohydrate, releasing methane gas in the process. If you have this problem, introduce more fiber into your diet slowly to determine what is a proper level for you. I do not usually recommend taking fiber supplements as pills, powders, or straight wheat bran. Not only can they give you gas, they can interfere with absorption of minerals from foods, and even impede bowel movements if you do not drink plenty of water with them. Just eat more fruits, vegetables, whole grains, seeds, and nuts, and you will have all the fiber in your diet you need.

PROTECTIVE PHYTOCHEMICALS

One of the most exciting areas of nutritional research today is identification and investigation of compounds in plants that can bolster our defenses against agents of disease, reducing risks of cancer and other serious illnesses. So many of these have come to light in recent years, with actions so varied and beneficial, that it is a wonder the consumption of fruits and vegetables is not going up faster than it is. You will find little or nothing about these phytochemicals in conventional nutrition textbooks and courses, but scientific papers about them are proliferating so rapidly that nutritionists will have to take note.

Strictly speaking, these micronutrients are not essential, in that the absence of them in the diet will not result in death or serious dysfunction. Nonetheless, I consider them vitally important, because our exposure to dangerous organisms and toxins has never been greater. To take just one example, living organisms have always had to deal with the oxidative stress of normal metabolism as well as oxidative pressures from the environment. To that background we have added tobacco smoke, air pollution, and a host of cancer-promoting chemicals in our water and food, some there by accident (industrial effluents) and some by design (pesticides on crops). It is likely that our natural antioxidant defenses—a large group of compounds, some made in the body, others provided by the diet, that work together to scavenge free radicals and block oxidation reactions—are overwhelmed and need all the help they can get.

Fortunately, many plants contain powerful antioxidants, in addition to the vitamins discussed above. One of the strongest and most studied is EGCG (epigallocatechin gallate) in green tea, which is also present in lesser amounts in apples. EGCG shows impressive activity against many kinds of cancer. It appears to protect the heart and arteries from oxidative damage, and, applied topically, may protect the skin from the damaging effects of ultraviolet radiation and reverse precancerous skin changes. You need to drink about four cups of green tea daily to get optimal doses of EGCG. Although green tea contains less caffeine than coffee, it is still a stimulant. So if you do not want to consume that much caffeine, you can get decaffeinated brands or take caffeine-free green-tea extracts as dietary supplements.

EGCG is one type of *catechin*. Catechins are condensed tannins, which, themselves, are one class of a larger group of protective phytochemicals called polyphenols. Polyphenols are widely distributed in nature, appearing in every plant family. They have powerful and varied anticancer activity and also protect against coronary heart disease. Polyphenols in extra-virgin olive oil protect its unsaturated fatty acids from oxidation and contribute to olive oil's health benefits.

Another class of antioxidant polyphenols found in many plants are red and purple pigments called anthocyanins and proanthocyanidins. They give color to berries, cherries, red grapes (and juice and wine made from them), plums, pomegranates, and red cabbage, and also

occur in some beans and grains. It is these pigments and their antioxidant effects, rather than alcohol, that mostly account for the cardiovascular benefits of red wine. You can get those benefits just as well
by drinking red grape juice or eating plenty of red and purple fruits.
The pigments in them protect hearts, lungs, and blood vessels from
degenerative changes.

The carotenoids, as mentioned above, are a different group of
antioxidant pigments. They give color to carrots, pumpkins, squash,
sweet potatoes, tomatoes, cantaloupes, peaches, mangos, and other
yellow and orange fruits and vegetables and are also abundant,
though not visible, in dark, leafy greens. We know that these fruits
and vegetables are strongly cancer-protective; we do not know that
any one member of the carotenoid family of pigments is chiefly
responsible for that protection.

A few years ago, beta carotene enjoyed a reputation as the number-
one carotenoid, and many people took it as a supplement, assuming
they were lowering their cancer risks by doing so. Then several well-
designed studies cast doubt on that assumption, even suggesting that
supplemental beta carotene might promote cancer in certain groups
(cigarette smokers, for one). Here hangs a cautionary tale. To recommend the use of one, isolated element of a complex family of protective compounds in plants is to fall under the spell of reductionism,
the belief that the part equals the whole. Unfortunately, that way of
thinking now dominates Western medicine and science.

It is the whole mix of carotenoids that confers protection from
cancer and degenerative disease, not any one of them. Lutein and
zeaxanthin appear to protect vision, lowering risks of developing
cataract and macular degeneration, the commonest causes of vision
loss in older people. Lycopene may reduce risks of prostate cancer.
Yet even a number of these brightly colored compounds in capsule
form may not be equal in effect to eating the fruits and vegetables
that contain them. I take a daily mixed carotenoid supplement for
insurance—for example, to cover those days when, for one reason or
another, I don't eat the appropriate foods. Still, I make an effort to
eat a rainbow mix of fresh fruits and vegetables and dark, leafy
greens, and I advise you to do the same.

Yet another category of protective phytochemicals are phytoestrogens, compounds in plants that can interact with estrogen receptors
on cells in the human body. This is a chemically diverse group,

including the isoflavones in soy and lignans in flax and other oil seeds. We still have a lot to learn about them and how they work. One theory is that phytoestrogens attach to estrogen receptors but activate them only weakly. Soy isoflavones may have enough estrogenic activity to prevent hot flashes in menopausal Japanese women, but by blocking access to the receptors they may also protect those women from other, stronger estrogenic agents, including environmental toxins and the growth-promoting hormones used in animals raised for food. They may also protect men from similar hormonal pressures on the prostate.

The epidemiological evidence for health-protective effects of soy is promising. Populations that eat a lot of it have low rates of breast cancer, menopausal problems, and prostate cancer. Still, there are many different phytoestrogens, and we do not know if all of them are protective or whether introducing them into the diet before puberty is wise or how they interact with prescribed hormones and drugs. As an example of the uncertainty, let me mention a kind of patient I see frequently: a woman with estrogen-receptor-positive breast cancer who is being treated with the estrogen-antagonist drug Tamoxifen following surgery. Tamoxifen can cause unpleasant side effects, including hot flashes. The patient finds that increasing her intake of soy foods mitigates the side effects of Tamoxifen. We do not know if it is also mitigating the therapeutic effects. The dose of soy might be critical. Some test-tube research suggests that low doses of soy isoflavones might stimulate cells with estrogen receptors to divide and proliferate, while higher doses might block them. Again, we don't know.

My guess is that the benefits of soy outweigh the risks. I also think one of the healthiest dietary changes Westerners could make would be to substitute soy foods for some of the animal foods they now eat. I believe that soy isoflavones can protect most people—men and women—from hormonally driven cancers as well as from coronary heart disease. They might even reduce the risk of osteoporosis.

One last group of phytochemicals I want you to be aware of are the polysaccharides in mushrooms. Polysaccharides are very large, long-chain sugar molecules that are structural components of many cells. They have never seemed terribly interesting to pharmacologists because they appear to be too big to be absorbed from the gut, are difficult to work with in the laboratory, and do not appear to be molecules that have therapeutic effects. Nonetheless, polysaccharides seem to be the active compounds in a number of medicinal plants and foods that are nontoxic but have powerful enhancing effects on immunity. They resemble constituents of bacterial cell walls and for that reason may be immunologically active. Macrophages—large, roving immune cells that leave blood vessels and move through tissues—can gobble up polysaccharides from the gut wall and transport them to other immune cells, initiating a chain of defensive events. This translates into increased numbers and activity of natural killer cells, which are the main destroyers of malignant cells, as well as increased resistance to invasion by bacteria and viruses.

These beneficial polysaccharides are not in the common button mushroom (*Agaricus bisporus*) popular in the West, but they are in a number of edible wild mushrooms and many of the species cultivated for food in Asia. Shiitake (*Lentinula edodes*), oyster mushrooms (*Pleurotus* spp.), enokidake (*Flammulina velutipes*), and maitake (*Grifola frondosa*) all contain them and make delicious additions to the diet. All of these mushrooms are becoming more available in our part of the world. It is worth getting to know them, not the least for their immune-enhancing qualities.

There are many other protective phytochemicals. There are ellagic acid in raspberries and blueberries, *d*-limonene in citrus peel, sulforaphane in broccoli, isothiocyanates in all the cabbage family vegetables—all potent cancer fighters. There is allicin in garlic, which lowers blood pressure and acts as a natural antibiotic. Ginger contains shogaols, which counter inflammation. Fruits and vegetables are loaded with protective phytochemicals. *Eat more fruits and vegetables.*

For every category of micronutrients—vitamins, minerals, fiber, and phytochemicals—my advice has been the same: increased consumption of fruits and vegetables. Nutritionists now recommend eating five to nine servings of these foods a day. A serving of fruit is one medium-sized piece or slice of melon; one-half cup of berries; one-half cup of canned fruit; one-quarter cup of dried fruit, or six ounces (three-quarters of a cup) of fruit juice. A serving of vegetables is one-half cup of chopped raw vegetables or the same amount of cooked (including cooked dried beans or lentils); one cup of leafy, raw vegetables; one medium potato; seven or eight carrot sticks, or six ounces of vegetable juice.

To give you an idea of how you might fit in nine servings over the course of a day, you might have a banana and a glass of orange juice at breakfast, two cups of salad and some vegetable juice at lunch, a cup of broccoli with dinner, and some berries and a slice of melon for dessert.

Fresh fruits and vegetables should be your first choice, because the content of nutrients is greater in fresh forms. Frozen fruits and vegetables are much better than canned. (I use some canned beans and tomatoes and keep a variety of berries in my freezer; otherwise I use only fresh produce.) Get the highest-quality fruits and vegetables you can, those that look attractive and are not old, tired, and discolored.

I have written elsewhere of the dangers of agrichemicals and of my strong belief in the importance of organic agriculture, which, I am happy to report, is growing exponentially, here and abroad. The quality and variety of organic produce are getting better and better. And as consumer demand increases, things can only continue to improve. Although organic produce is becoming available in more and more supermarkets, I am aware that it is still difficult for many people to find, and it is more expensive than conventional produce. One strategy for dealing with this situation is to learn which crops are most likely to carry unhealthful residues of pesticides and fungicides and to avoid them or minimize consumption if you cannot find organic versions.

The list of suspect crops changes over time, but strawberries always top it. They are often full of methyl bromide, a fungicide and known carcinogen, that consumer pressure has so far been unsuccessful in eliminating, and I do not eat them if I cannot find organically grown ones. Quite recently, the availability of organic strawberries increased dramatically in America. They are much more flavorful than conventional strawberries (and also spoil more quickly). Other regulars on the most contaminated list are peaches, apricots, cherries, grapes from Chile, Mexican cantaloupes, green beans, celery, and spinach. I also recommend trying to eat only organic potatoes and wheat (including flour).

I always wash produce before using it. If you use conventionally grown fruits and vegetables, it is especially important to wash them carefully and peel them when appropriate. A 1996 study done at the

Southwestern Research Institute in San Antonio, Texas, tested seventeen different fruits and vegetables and found that washing (and peeling) removed all traces of pesticides from more than half the samples with detectable residues and significantly lowered signs of them in the rest.

The researchers used the following washing method: They swirled grapes, berries, green beans, and leafy vegetables (outer leaves removed) in a dilute solution of dish detergent and room-temperature water—about one teaspoon of detergent per gallon—for five to ten seconds, then rinsed them with warm water. They scrubbed the sturdier fruits and vegetables with the same solution, using a vegetable brush, then rinsed them the same way. Peeling was enough to get rid of all residues in acorn squash, bananas, and corn on the cob, while scrubbing, rinsing, and peeling removed all residues from carrots and potatoes. Peeling is especially important to remove fungicides from fruits and vegetables that are waxed, such as cucumbers and apples.

Eating more fruits and vegetables, in whatever form, is clearly an excellent way to improve your diet and take advantage of the healing properties of food.

A HEALING STORY:
A SUCCESSFUL ENCOUNTER
WITH INTEGRATIVE MEDICINE

WHEN SHE was forty-nine and working as a coordinator in the College of Architecture at the University of Arizona, Karen Young was treated at the Integrative Medicine Clinic at the University Medical Center. For many years she had suffered from irritable bowel syndrome, for which she had found no relief despite numerous visits to internists and gastroenterologists. She recalls:

I developed some sort of fatigue syndrome. If I stayed up late, my hands and limbs would swell, and I got very tired. It was a mystery disease. One rheumatologist told me it could be scleroderma or lupus. I'd always thought of myself as a high-energy kind of person, so this was a real problem.

From the beginning, my experience in the clinic was wonderful. Dr. Victoria Maizes spent an hour and a half with me on the first visit, taking my history more thoroughly than anyone ever had: my lifestyle, including my diet, my attitude toward work, and so forth. I had been a vegetarian for a long time, then had started to eat meat. I was always thin, so I could eat whatever I wanted, which probably didn't serve me well as I got older. I was in the habit of drinking a lot of Coca-Cola, though I never thought of myself as a user of caffeine.

Dr. Maizes noticed my habit of chewing on the inside of my mouth. I do this a lot when I'm at work. It's a stupid habit that makes my mouth sore. I tried to deal with it by chewing sugarless gum instead, which I did very often. Dr. Maizes told me that sugarless gum is not good for irritable bowel syndrome. [The nonabsorbable sugars xylitol and sorbitol in the gum draw water into the gut, increasing its activity.] I quit it, as she had recommended, and it made an enormous difference for the better. No doctor I had seen ever told me this or even asked about whether I used sugarless products.

Dr. Maizes also suggested that I drink green tea. I had never tried it. I now drink two cups of green tea a day, and that has also made a big difference. It gives me energy but calms me at the same time. I always carry a bag of it with me and take a supply when I travel. I now drink hot tea instead of a Coke. In fact I'm not drinking any carbonated soft drinks. I think stopping all that sugar intake was significant.

My husband and I recently remodeled our kitchen and took the opportunity to put in a water purification system. And I've improved my diet steadily. I now eat little red meat. I eat salmon twice a week. I've always loved vegetables more than anything.

I hardly have irritable bowel symptoms any more—a remarkable difference. My energy is great. I don't know if it's just the diet or the whole feeling I got in the clinic. It's wonderful to feel I have control over my own well-being. That alone has made me feel more empowered and positive. I wish everyone could experience this kind of medicine!

A HEALING STORY:
OVERCOMING ALLERGIES

ELIZABETH TRATTNER is now thirty-five years old and the mother of a very healthy two-year-old named Charlotte. Once a professional model, Elizabeth now practices Chinese medicine in south Florida. Ten years ago, when she came to me as a patient, she was suffering from severe, chronic asthma, sinusitis, and allergies—so severe that she had often been hospitalized and was dependent on high-dose steroids. Here is her story:

Allergies run in my family. I was not breastfed as a baby; instead I was given formula containing Karo syrup and soy. I was lactose intolerant, but no one knew that—my parents thought I was just prone to gas and stomachaches—and throughout childhood I drank a lot of milk. In my teenage years I suffered intense menstrual cramps and was always tired and congested, though I never had sinus or ear infections.

Through my college years I often got sick. Whenever I ate dairy products I would soon have crippling bouts of diarrhea accompanied by hot flashes and cold sweats. By my senior year I had given up most dairy products, because I knew they were making me sick. But by then my immune system was going haywire. I had lost fifteen pounds and was suffering from asthma. I gave up *all* dairy, including products containing whey and casein. By then, I had also developed a bad allergy to wheat. Soon I had to give up oranges and all fruits and vegetables in the squash family, as well as most processed foods, whose additives bothered me. If I ate foods that I was sensitive to, I would vomit. I kept getting sicker; at one point I spent a hundred days in the hospital and could eat only carrots, oatmeal, and brown rice.

I learned that many doctors don't believe in food allergies and that the skin tests allergists administer don't show how your gut reacts. I had to learn to solve my health problems on my own. For instance, I became aware of the dangers of sulfites [a class of preservatives] when I went into anaphylactic shock on an airplane after eating a snack of golden raisins. (Balsamic vinegar contains sulfites, too.)

But all was not lost. I learned to eat very well—that was the silver lining in all of this. I tried to eat organic produce as much as possible and was able to introduce new foods gradually. Today I feel better than I have in a long time. As long as I eat well, I feel clearheaded, not tired, and not congested. After twelve years on steroids, I stopped taking them in April 1999. But I'm still so sensitive that if I go out and have even one meal of bad food, I feel horrible the next day, like a hangover.

My daughter Charlotte is a fabulous and most unusual eater. While I was pregnant I stuffed myself with salmon and other essential fatty acid sources in the last trimester and breastfed her for six months. She has never had dairy in her life. She loves rice noodles for breakfast. I restrict her wheat. She eats all green vegetables, loves green beans with garlic and olive oil, and hates sweets. She actually refuses cookies offered to her and seems to prefer salty rice crackers and bitter drinks, like unsweetened green tea. She doesn't much like juice. I give her organic turkey and chicken and fish; she doesn't like red meat. She likes dark chocolate in small amounts but refuses milk chocolate. She loves seeds and nuts (but not peanuts), eats kale—can you believe it?—and loves rice. The only thing bad she eats is French fries. She's almost never sick. And I'm a happy mom.

3

THE WORST DIET
IN THE WORLD

NOW THAT you understand the basics of human nutrition and the role of macronutrients and micronutrients in the diet, I would like you to try a little thought experiment with me. Using the information in the last chapter, let's put our heads together to see if we can design the Worst Diet in the World, one that would be most likely to undermine health and shorten life.

To begin, let's stuff it with calories, more than most people will be able to burn off, so that it will promote obesity. In particular, we should overload it with carbohydrate calories from high-glycemic-index foods. That means lots of refined flour in fluffy breads and pastries, a lot of potatoes, sweets, and sweet drinks—fruit juices and sodas—especially those made with high-fructose corn syrup to take advantage of any disruptive effects of that product on metabolism.

For fat we will need a glut of saturated fat in the form of cheese, butter, cream, and other whole-milk products, along with a lot of beef and unskinned chicken. That will ensure that most people will develop unhealthy levels of serum cholesterol and increased risks of cardiovascular disease. We should also include plenty of hydrogenated fat in the form of margarine, vegetable shortening, and snack foods made with partially hydrogenated oils. And why don't we include refined, polyunsaturated vegetable oils for their carcinogenic potential and ability to damage cellular structures and accelerate aging? By doing so, we can move the ratio of omega-6 to omega-3 fatty acids in our diet further in the wrong direction. We should also throw in some well-used cooking fat, consisting of cheaper vegetable oils, to get even more *trans*-fatty acids and their damaging effects on membranes, hormones, and cardiovascular function. (Deep-fried Mars bars?)

As for protein, we should probably go for as much as we can eat and make it mostly commercially raised meat and poultry rather than fish or vegetable protein. That will maximize intake of drugs and hormones used to raise animals for meat as well as environmental toxins concentrated in their fat and other tissues. A lot of the meat in the diet should be processed (into hot dogs, lunch meats, and the like) to add more sodium, saturated fat, and unhealthful chemical additives. We should encourage everyone to drink cow's milk throughout life to make sure we affect the lactose-intolerant fraction of the population, aggravate allergy and autoimmunity, and get more butterfat into people's systems for good atherogenic measure.

The Worst Diet in the World should also be distinguished by what it does not provide. We will want very inadequate amounts of the micronutrients, especially those that protect the body from effects we are trying to achieve by the above selection of macronutrients. The easiest way to make sure of that is to restrict fruits and vegetables. Of course, we will allow unrestricted amounts of floury potatoes (preferably French fried or otherwise prepared with quantities of margarine, butter, and sour cream) and refined grains for their high-glycemic impact, but we don't want people eating too many greens and brightly colored fruits and vegetables. We can let them have canned fruit in heavy syrup and maybe some conventional strawberries for a dollop of pesticide residues now and then, but they ought to keep their vegetable consumption down to some iceberg lettuce smothered in dressing made from unhealthful fat and maybe corn on the cob with lots of butter. Perhaps pickles, high in sodium, and ketchup, high in sugar and sodium, will count as vegetables in our diet. These rules will keep fiber intake low, prevent people from eating too many protective phytochemicals, and maybe even get levels of vitamins and minerals down low enough to cause suboptimal functioning of many systems of the body without producing overt deficiency symptoms that might lead people to take corrective action.

From what I know about the scientific basis of human nutrition, I am quite sure that a diet of this sort, though it will sustain life and growth, will also have tremendous consequences as people age. It will increase the frequency of degenerative diseases, lowering the age at which they appear, accelerating their progression, and worsening their severity. It will certainly promote obesity, hypertension, coronary heart disease, and cancer and probably will adversely affect liver, kidney, and brain function. By impairing immunity and the healing response, it should increase susceptibility to infection and toxic injury. By promoting inflammation, it may increase the incidence of arthritis, bursitis, tendinitis, and the general aches and pains of aging. It might even make people less energetic and worsen their moods.

Thus we will have more than accomplished our goal.

Thank you for indulging this exercise in fantasy. Now I have a real-world assignment for you. I would like you to visit three different fast-food restaurants of your choice, study the menus in them, and observe what the customers are eating. Then I want you to think about how closely those menus approximate the Worst Diet in the World we have just designed.

Fast food has been one of the most unhealthful dietary developments in human history. It is mostly an American invention of the late twentieth century, one that we are now busily exporting all over the world. Of course, people love fast food, especially kids. Already, it has changed the eating habits of a large and growing fraction of the population.

Fast food is so attractive primarily because it caters to inherited tastes for fat, animal protein, and sugar, and the learned taste for salt. It is also convenient and predictable.

The tastiness of fast food must be acknowledged. Obviously, burgers, fries, milk shakes, and cola appeal to many people in many cultures; witness the wild success of American fast-food chains in Japan, China, Russia, and Latin America. The combination of appealing taste, attractive packaging, and clever marketing is powerful. I find it most distressing that people with access to more healthful dietary choices turn so readily to fast food when it becomes available.

The convenience of fast food is clearly one of its major selling points. In our society, many people no longer have time to prepare meals, let alone wash, cut, and cook fresh vegetables. In families where both parents work, time is short, and since kids love fast food, it becomes a very tempting option.

The predictability of fast food appears to be a source of comfort and reassurance to many in our highly mobile, fast-paced culture. The sight of a familiar sign or logo of a fast-food restaurant means respite from the road and the uncertainties of travel. There will be no surprises inside. It is always the same menu, with the food prepared the same way, looking and tasting the same. There will be no strange foods to scare the kids, nothing that stretches the experience of eating. Personally, I find this aspect of fast food depressing. Having started to travel at a young age, I always looked forward to novelty and surprise, especially at the table. For me, one of the great delights of visiting other cultures is trying new food. So it used to be in traveling around the United States in the days before interstate highways, malls, and shopping centers, all with totally predictable food choices.

I want people to change their eating habits to improve health, and I am especially concerned about the eating habits of children, because they often persist throughout life. I am also aware that unless healthful food meets the standards of taste, convenience, and reassurance provided by fast food, it stands little chance of gaining ground.

At the beginning of this book I stated as one of my basic principles of diet and health: Food that is healthy and food that gives pleasure are not mutually exclusive. I stand by that statement. And I keep waiting for some bright, aware entrepreneur with the necessary business and marketing skills to open a chain of healthful fast-food restaurants. They would have to offer all the taste, convenience, and comfort of existing establishments while following the basic principles set forth in this book. I know that such an enterprise is possible and would be successful. I would gladly lend my support to it.

A Healing Story:
Learning to Make
Healthful Food

EVER SINCE I've known her, Wendy Kohatsu, M.D., has been a conscious eater of healthful food, but she says she wasn't always. One of the first physicians to graduate from the Program in Integrative Medicine at the University of Arizona, Wendy is now an assistant professor of family and community medicine at East Tennessee State University and a strong proponent of nutritional medicine. She is a fourth-generation Japanese-American who grew up in Los Angeles as a "total carnivore," but she changed her diet while in college as a result of having a vegetarian boyfriend.

"I switched to a vegetarian diet as an experiment, not intending to stay on it," she recalls, "but not eating meat agreed with me. I also cut out most dairy products, which I think I'm not genetically equipped to digest." She now eats a lot of vegetables, soy foods, whole grains, fruits, and some fish, and is especially careful to get adequate amounts of omega-3 fatty acids. She makes herself a smoothie every morning with flax oil as an omega-3 source.

"After about a year of eating this way," says Wendy, "I got a massage from a therapist who asked whether I was a vegetarian. I asked him how he knew. He said he could tell from the consistency of my flesh—that it was different from that of a meat-eater. I found that remarkable."

While in residency training at the University of California and San Francisco General Hospital, Wendy assisted in some of the group programs given by Dr. Dean Ornish for patients wanting to reverse heart disease through lifestyle change. This experience strengthened her interest in motivating patients to change their eating habits in order to improve their health. She tells the following story:

In 1997, in my last year of training, along with two other family practice residents, I created a wellness class for patients based on the Ornish philosophy. The goal was to teach people how to eat better as well as to help them reduce stress through education and group support. The class met on Tuesday nights for three hours over eight weeks, and we gave it twice, once in winter, once in spring, with about eight participants each time. The patients mostly had heart disease, hypertension, obesity, and related disorders— similar to those I worked with in the Ornish programs—but the demographics were very different. Ornish attracted mostly affluent, educated white people. About 80 percent of our groups were minorities from underserved populations. Most were African American or Hispanic.

The work was psychologically challenging. With the Ornish groups, I could talk about the latest research on antioxidants. Now I had to answer such questions as "Is the white or yellow part of the egg the bad part?" And when I tried to talk about the importance of exercise, I got responses like "I'd like to walk, but there's too much gang violence in my neighborhood."

We decided to teach very basic nutrition. One strategy was to ask people to talk about their favorite foods and think about how to make more healthful versions of them. We thought this would be more realistic than trying to turn these people into vegetarians. We planned a potluck for the last evening of the course, where people could bring in their dishes and discuss the recipes.

I remember especially a Salvadoran woman named Rosa, who had told us that her favorite food was fried plaintains, the big, starchy bananas of the tropics. Usually, thick slices of the fruit are fried in large amounts of oil till golden, often pressed into patties with a fork. Rosa said these were a staple at family meals. We helped her figure out a better way to cook them, and she brought a big dish of the new version to the potluck. With great enthusiasm she explained that she left the skin on and poked holes in it to let the steam out. Then she baked the plaintains in the oven for an hour. After that she peeled and sliced them and browned the slices in just a bit of oil. She told the group proudly that her family liked these just as much as the ones she used to make.

I now work in a rural area of eastern Tennessee, where the local diet is not terrific. Every time I have a chance, I talk to patients about how they eat and give them practical suggestions for making changes for the better. And I'm committed to making nutrition a central aspect of the medicine of the future.

4

THE BEST DIET
IN THE WORLD

YOU CAN EASILY construct the Best Diet in the World, in general terms at least, by simply writing down the contrary of the principles we just used to design a wretched diet and by following the recommendations I gave you at the ends of the sections about carbohydrate, fat, protein, and micronutrients. Rather than repeat those recommendations, I would like to approach the subject by examining a number of very different diets that experts, including some nutritionists and physicians, have advanced as candidates for the title of Best Diet in the World. Later (Appendix A), I will give you my recommendations for the optimum diet.

THE PALEOLITHIC DIET

Let's start with prehistory and look again at the Paleolithic diet. Some experts say that if we ate like our distant hunter-gatherer ancestors most of our health problems, including obesity and cardiovascular disease, would disappear.

As noted earlier the Paleolithic diet contained no processed food and very little carbohydrate, since agriculture to produce grains had not yet been invented. It included a lot of meat from wild game, fish, some wild fruits, nuts, and tubers but few vegetables and no salt or vegetable oils. To my mind, the main advantages of this diet are:

- no processed foods (with their unhealthful forms of carbohydrate and fat and a high content of additives)

- meat and fowl with lower and more healthful fat content than modern versions and none of their residues of drugs and hormones
- a very favorable omega-6 to omega-3 ratio in the range of two to one or one to one
- some wild seeds and nuts to provide fiber and micronutrients
- none of the high-glycemic carbohydrate load of the modern diet

The drawbacks of this diet are:

- insufficient carbohydrate for continuous maintenance of glycogen stores
- insufficient fruits and vegetables to provide fiber and micronutrients, especially protective phytochemicals
- excessive animal protein with its consequent strain on liver and kidney function

Bottom line: Few people in Paleolithic times lived long enough to develop the degenerative diseases that afflict human beings today. It is unrealistic to expect people to give up carbohydrate staples like bread and pasta; the task is to persuade them to eat smaller amounts of carbohydrate and better forms of it, with lower glycemic index. I don't see the fast-food restaurant of tomorrow serving Paleolithic cuisine. What we should chiefly borrow from this diet are its absence of processed food and its desirable ratio of omega-6 to omega-3 fatty acids.

THE RAW FOODS DIET

If food processing is the problem, some say, why not go back even further in time to before the invention of cooking? A diet of all raw foods would certainly be more natural; it is, after all, the way wild animals eat. We know that cooking can destroy some micronutrients (when you boil foods containing water-soluble vitamins, you lose them unless you also consume the water) and create toxins (blackened animal flesh is carcinogenic). A number of doctors and clinics urge people who are ailing to eat only raw foods to regain their health, and I have visited raw-food restaurants in several American cities. These are purely vegetarian, of course. Possible advantages of this way of eating include:

- plenty of fruits, vegetables, seeds, and nuts and their content of micronutrients
- no chance of fiber deficiency
- little processed food
- no flesh foods with the contaminants they may contain
- little danger of getting too much protein or fat or the wrong kind of fat

And the disadvantages:

- loss of much of the best flavor, texture, and appearance of food
- low bioavailability of many micronutrients
- too many natural toxins in raw vegetables

Bottom line: These last two points require some explanation. The vitamins and minerals in raw vegetables may be much less available to the body than those in cooked vegetables. For example, the body cannot obtain lycopene, the carotenoid pigment that protects against prostate cancer, from raw tomatoes, only from cooked ones and then only if fat is present in the digestive tract to facilitate absorption. (A fragrant marinara sauce made with olive oil is a perfect lycopene source.*) Similarly, all the carotenoids in carrots become much more available to the body when you cook the carrots. That does not mean you should not eat raw carrots; it does mean you should eat some cooked carrots, say in soup, stews, or stir-fries.

As for natural toxins in vegetables, I have written on this subject before but still find that many people are uninformed about it. Some roots, seeds, stems, and leaves contain natural toxins, most of which are destroyed by simple cooking. Most raw beans are in this category, along with their sprouts. Alfalfa sprouts, much loved by raw-food enthusiasts, are full of canavanine, a natural toxin that can harm the immune system. Common button mushrooms contain agaritine, a natural carcinogen. Celery tends to produce psoralens, compounds that sensitize the skin to the harmful effects of ultraviolet radiation in sunlight. Our bodies have defenses against toxins in food we eat, but those defenses are overwhelmed these days; it cannot do

*A recipe is on page 242.

any good to add to the total toxic load they have to deal with. The occurrence of natural toxins in common edible plants and the great potential of cooking to neutralize them is a good argument against eating nothing but raw foods.

THE TRADITIONAL JAPANESE DIET

Until recently, the Japanese were the healthiest people on the planet. They are still the nation with the greatest longevity: an average of 77.2 years for men and 84.1 years for women, but in 1998, the Japan Hospital Association, which has been surveying overall health of those Japanese undergoing full physical examinations since 1984, reported that the percentage of healthy people dropped to a fifteen-year low. The report attributed the decline to rising blood cholesterol levels and alcohol-related liver problems and noted a long-term change in Japanese food tastes from the traditional, healthful diet of fish, vegetables, and rice to fast foods, meat, and bread. This change has also caused rates of obesity to rise.

Even if most Japanese no longer eat the traditional Japanese diet, it is worth looking at because of its close correlation with very low rates of coronary heart disease and of hormonally driven cancers so prevalent in the West. This diet is very distinctive, including foods and preparations of foods not found elsewhere in the world. Its advantages are:

- an unusually low percentage of total calories from fat—about 10 percent—for a cuisine that so many people find appetizing and interesting
- lots of fresh fish but very little meat and no milk or milk products
- high omega-3 fatty acid intake as a result of emphasis on fish and sea vegetables
- astonishing variety and a vast range of colors, flavors (including bitter), and textures of food
- inclusion of a great many fresh vegetables, both raw and cooked (and pickled)
- inclusion of many types of soy foods on a daily basis
- few sweets, except for fruit in season, and little use of sugar except in small amounts as a seasoning
- little use of wheat flour or other forms of finely particulate starch,

except in noodles that are generally eaten hot or cold in low-fat broths rather than high-fat sauces

- inclusion of many wild foods, including vegetables, sea vegetables, and mushrooms
- an emphasis on the aesthetics of food and food preparation that make it the most artistic cuisine in the world
- an emphasis on seasonality—eating foods in season and harmonizing qualities of dishes with the qualities of the season
- consciousness of the impact of food on health, both preventively and therapeutically
- inclusion of green tea, with its powerful antioxidant effects

As for the drawbacks of this diet, I would list:

- many ingredients and foods too strange for Western tastes
- the need for a great deal of time and work to prepare most dishes and meals
- very high salt content, related to use of shoyu (soy sauce), miso (fermented soybean paste), and pickled vegetables, all containing much added salt, and sea vegetables with naturally high sodium content—these foods present at every meal
- low content of the specific kind of fiber from bran as a result of preference for polished (white) rice

Bottom line: The traditional Japanese diet is associated with great longevity and low incidence of "Western" diseases. It could be improved by decreasing its salt content and adding unpolished rice. Unfortunately, this cuisine cannot easily be exported except to Japanese restaurants. It is too labor intensive and time consuming—the quintessential "slow food"—and it includes too many items, textures, and flavors that do not appeal to non-Japanese. Nonetheless, it seems very worthwhile trying to incorporate into an optimum diet some of the principles of the traditional Japanese diet.

For example, the principles of variety, food aesthetics, seasonality, and desirability of wild foods are important and adaptable to other cuisines. I have already stated my belief that low-meat, low-milk, high-fish consumption is better than the Western pattern of protein intake. Despite its reliance on white rice, the traditional Japanese diet's carbohydrate profile is not associated with the kinds of problems associated with carbohydrates in the Western diet, especially obesity.

THE "ASIAN DIET"

I see much in print these days about the health benefits of the Asian diet, even an Asian Food Pyramid as an alternative to the usual U.S. Department of Agriculture diagram with its recommended intakes of various food groups. The problem is that there is no general Asian diet. The different nations of the Far East eat very different kinds of food. For example, Chinese cuisine is nothing like Japanese, since it features mostly cooked food instead of raw and much more animal protein. In northern China, people eat as much wheat as rice. Koreans eat more meat still, especially barbecued beef, and a great deal of strong spices like ginger, garlic, and chile. Thais eat fiery curries cooked in coconut milk, a lot of tropical fruit, and more sweets than East Asians. Vietnamese cuisine is heavily influenced by French cooking, as a result of the former French colonial presence. Indonesian food includes elaborate curries and such unique ingredients as tempeh, a fermented soy product. Indians, distinct from other Asians, use dairy products in the form of fresh cheese, yogurt, and butter; they also like sweets very much and use a cornucopia of spices. In the south of India, where orthodox Hinduism prevails, the diet is lacto-vegetarian. In the north, where Muslim influence is strong, people eat a lot of beef and lamb.

So it seems to me risky to try to draw generalizations from such a mix, but I think that when people in the West talk about the advantages of the Asian diet, they mean a plant-based diet that includes relatively little meat, poultry, and sweets. Its advantages are:

- lots of vegetables and fruits
- fewer refined carbohydrates and less sugar than the Western diet provides
- less and more healthful fat
- less meat and milk and more fish than in the Western diet
- high flavor appeal through the artful use of herbs and spices
- inclusion of soy foods
- relatively few processed foods
- tea as the main beverage, with its antioxidant effects

Of course, these are all features I would like to keep in an optimum diet for people in our society. The disadvantages of the Asian diet, as you might expect, are:

- too much salt
- many unfamiliar ingredients
- labor-intensive food preparation
- unhealthful fat (refined vegetable oils, coconut oil, and coconut milk, depending on the particular cuisine)
- too much animal protein, depending on the particular cuisine

Bottom line: Westerners are learning to like Asian food. Two of the most popular restaurant styles in America at the moment are "Pacific Rim" and "Asian Fusion," in which chefs often apply cooking methods and flavor principles of Far Eastern cooking to Western foods. They produce much more interesting and more healthful dishes than those served at usual Western restaurants. The questions are whether this kind of food lends itself to home preparation and whether large numbers of Westerners would ever eat it on a regular basis.

THE VEGAN DIET

A minority of physicians urge people to eschew all animal foods— milk, milk products, and eggs as well as flesh foods. They may have been drawn to this way of eating by spiritual or ethical considerations but now try to rationalize their food choices in medical terms. Vegan food can be either boring or delicious, depending on the creativity and sensitivity of the cook. Many Westerners forced to eat this way would probably lose weight, have better serum lipid profiles, and lower risks of chronic disease for obvious reasons. They would be consuming less fat, less saturated fat, less animal protein, and more fruits and vegetables than before, all changes in the right direction. A recent small study of adult-onset diabetic patients found greater weight loss and improvement of blood sugar levels in those who followed a low-fat vegan diet for twelve weeks than in those on a conventional low-fat diet.

The advantages of a diet devoid of animal foods are:

- much less saturated fat and cholesterol than in a conventional diet
- much higher content of fruits and vegetables
- lower intake of environmental toxins

The disadvantages are:

- lack of appeal for most people
- risk of vitamin B$_{12}$ deficiency without adequate supplementation
- increased risk of omega-3 fatty acid deficiency (especially of EPA and DHA)
- increased risk of iron and calcium deficiency unless foods rich in usable forms of these minerals are emphasized or supplementation is provided

Bottom line: In my experience, most Westerners like artfully prepared vegan dishes but are unlikely to eat them exclusively. It is useful to know that one can make tasty food without using animal products, and I have already given my strong recommendation that you try to reduce the percentage of animal foods in your diet. But I do not see vegan cuisine becoming widely accepted in our society.

THE MEDITERRANEAN DIET

Perhaps the most talked-about diet in recent years is a composite of the cuisines of Spain, southern France, Italy, Greece, Crete, and parts of the Middle East. One of the first American experts to draw attention to the healthful qualities of diets in these countries was Ancel Keys, Ph.D., a physiologist who founded the Laboratory of Physiological Hygiene at the University of Minnesota in 1940. Keys developed the notorious K-ration for U.S. military troops in World War II and pioneered the investigation of the relationship between dietary fat, serum cholesterol, and the risk of coronary heart disease. His book, *Eat Well, Stay Well the Mediterranean Way,* published in 1975, is now out of print.

The best-known contemporary champion of the Mediterranean diet is Walter Willett, Ph.D., chairman of the department of nutrition at the Harvard School of Public Health and coinvestigator on the Harvard Nurses' Study. He is the developer of the Mediterranean Diet Pyramid, which emphasizes olive oil, fish above meat, and cheese above milk. Willett is also the most prominent nutritional authority urging us to pay more attention to the kind of fat in the diet as a determinant of health rather than simply the amount. As might be expected, he has drawn criticism from advocates of very low fat diets, who are upset with the Mediterranean Diet Pyramid because it

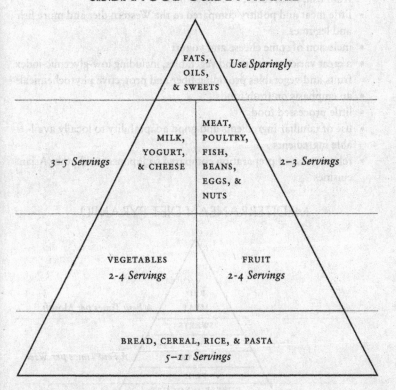

U.S.D.A. FOOD GUIDE PYRAMID

FATS, OILS, & SWEETS — *Use Sparingly*

MILK, YOGURT, & CHEESE — *3–5 Servings*

MEAT, POULTRY, FISH, BEANS, EGGS, & NUTS — *2–3 Servings*

VEGETABLES — *2-4 Servings*

FRUIT — *2-4 Servings*

BREAD, CEREAL, RICE, & PASTA — *5–11 Servings*

fails to tell people to cut their total fat intake. The U.S.D.A. Food Guide Pyramid puts fats and oils at the very top along with sweets with a cautionary note to "Use Sparingly." In the Mediterranean Diet Pyramid, red meat is at the very top, and a whole middle layer is devoted to olive oil, placed just above a thick layer of fruits, vegetables, and beans and nuts.

The plusses of the Mediterranean diet are:

- great variety and tastes that appeal to people of many different cultures
- lots of whole-grain products as opposed to refined carbohydrates in the Western diet, hence a reduced glycemic load

- mostly monounsaturated fat and plenty of omega-3 fatty acids from fish, nuts, seeds, and vegetables
- little meat and poultry compared to the Western diet and more fish and legumes
- inclusion of some cheese and yogurt
- a great variety of fruits and vegetables, including low-glycemic-index fruits and vegetables providing fiber and protective phytochemicals
- an emphasis on fresh foods
- little processed food
- use of familiar ingredients and good adaptability to locally available ingredients
- relative ease of preparation compared to Japanese and other Asian cuisines

MEDITERRANEAN DIET PYRAMID

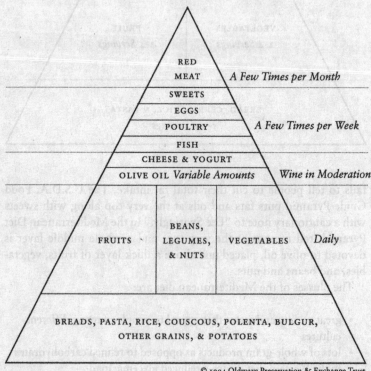

RED MEAT — *A Few Times per Month*

SWEETS
EGGS
POULTRY — *A Few Times per Week*
FISH

CHEESE & YOGURT
OLIVE OIL *Variable Amounts* — *Wine in Moderation*

FRUITS   BEANS, LEGUMES, & NUTS   VEGETABLES — *Daily*

BREADS, PASTA, RICE, COUSCOUS, POLENTA, BULGUR, OTHER GRAINS, & POTATOES

© 1994 Oldways Preservation & Exchange Trust

The drawbacks of this diet are very few:

- may not provide enough iron for growing children and pregnant women, unless iron-rich foods are emphasized
- may not provide enough calcium unless calcium-rich foods are emphasized or supplemental calcium is added

Bottom line: With few exceptions, the Mediterranean diet comes very close to adhering to all of the nutritional recommendations I have given you as well as to conforming to all of the basic principles of eating well I wrote about in the first chapter of this book. It is a style of eating that I like very much and one associated with much lower incidence of obesity, cardiovascular disease, and cancer than in most of Europe and the Americas. And it is certainly a cuisine that offers much delight for the senses, not at all a cuisine of deprivation.

I do want to point out a few cautions about unbridled enthusiasm for the Mediterranean diet. In the first place, I am speaking about the traditional Mediterranean diet, which may be starting to go the way of the traditional Japanese diet. In Greece, Italy, and Spain, processed food and American fast food are appearing as they are everywhere, and affluence brings with it greater consumption of calories and meat. Also, the traditional Mediterranean diet exists in a particular cultural context, in which people get more physical activity than most Americans and enjoy strong social and family bonds around meals. Eating together and taking pleasure in food are central to these healthy societies. It's not just the olive oil.

I hope these analyses of diets will help you design your own diet for optimum health. Keep in mind that there is no one right way to eat and that your nutritional needs may change over time. It is possible to adapt the principles of healthful eating presented in this book to a wide range of styles of food preparation, from Chinese to Italian. Eating well does not mean giving up everything you like. Even occasional self-indulgence in less healthful foods is not a disaster, and any steps you take to remedy what you are now doing wrong are steps in the right direction. Eating well simply means using a basic understanding of human nutrition to maximize as much as you can both the nourishing and pleasure-giving qualities of food.

As examples of how the common attributes of good diets from around the world can be put together into a practical, realistic plan, here is a week's worth of menus to give you a sense of what *Eating Well for Optimum Health* might look like in action. You will find recipes for starred items in the recipe section that begins on page 209. I offer these as examples of balanced meals that conform to the dietary guidelines in this book. Feel free to design your own.

BREAKFASTS

- a cup of berries, high-fiber cereal with soy milk
- fresh fruit, smoked salmon on whole-grain toast
- fresh fruit, scrambled eggs or tofu, whole-grain toast
- fruit juice, a whole-grain waffle with fruit spread, tofu sausages
- fresh fruit with nonfat yogurt, Banana Bread* or Pumpkin Muffin*
- fresh fruit, oatmeal with soy milk
- fresh fruit, toasted whole-grain bread with almond butter

LUNCHES

- soy or grain burger on whole-grain bun with lettuce and tomato, cole slaw
- a bowl of Mushroom Barley Soup* and a mixed green salad with olive oil and vinegar dressing
- Lentil Salad* with whole-grain bread
- Sardine or Kipper Sandwich Spread* on whole-grain bread with lettuce and tomato
- Pasta with Marinara Sauce* and Parmesan cheese, mixed green salad with olive oil and vinegar dressing
- Pasta Fagiole* (white bean and pasta soup), whole-grain crackers, an apple or pear
- Hummus* with whole-wheat pita bread and Middle Eastern Chopped Salad*

DINNERS

- Easy Poached Salmon* with Cranberry Wheatberry Salad*, steamed broccoli (with olive oil and garlic, if desired); fresh fruit or Blueberry Pie* for dessert
- Pasta with Kale*, a large mixed green salad with olive oil and vinegar dressing; fresh fruit or fruit sorbet for dessert

- Roasted Vegetable Soup*, baked beans with tofu wieners, Orange-Jicama Salad*; berries for dessert
- Asparagus Soup*, Dill-Poached Fish Fillets* with Tartar Sauce*, Couscous*, and a mixed green salad with olive oil and vinegar dressing; Raspberry Chocolate Pie* for dessert
- Stir-Fried Rice*, Green Cabbage and Mushrooms*; Carrot Cake* for dessert
- Soy or grain burgers on whole-wheat buns, Oven-Fried Potatoes*, Sweet-and-Sour Stir-Fried Red Cabbage; fresh fruit for dessert
- Quick Creamy Tomato Soup*, Mediterranean Tuna Steaks*, Robust Beet Salad*; fresh fruit and Cookies* for dessert

SNACKS

- Carrot sticks, a small handful of raw pumpkin seeds or nuts, a piece of natural cheese with rye crispbread, an apple, a piece of dark chocolate

BEVERAGES

- Pure water is your best bet. Mineral water, with or without gas, is also acceptable. I encourage the regular consumption of tea, hot or iced, with green tea preferred for its cancer- and heart-protective effects. Decaffeinated forms are available if you do not want to ingest caffeine. Wine in moderation is also all right, preferably not every day. Red wine has significant antioxidant activity, and additive-free, organic brands are becoming more available.

These suggested menus assume that you have the interest and time to prepare meals from scratch. The recipes at the end of this book are easy and quick to make; nevertheless, I recognize that many readers may take many of their meals at restaurants. Let me give you a week's worth of restaurant lunches and dinners that will also give you the benefits of eating well for optimum health.

LUNCHES

- Vegetable soup and a tuna sandwich on whole-grain bread
- A large salad of mixed greens with olive oil and vinegar and cheese (blue, Swiss, or goat)
- Beans and rice with a small salad

- Your favorite sushi with an order of *edamame* and green tea
- Pasta with marinara sauce and a small salad
- Fresh-fruit plate with low-fat cottage cheese
- Stir-fried vegetables with rice (with tofu if possible)

DINNERS

- Salad, spaghetti with olive oil and garlic (*aglio e olio*)
- Broiled salmon with vegetables and rice
- Vegetable antipasto; pasta with tomatoes, basil, and Parmesan cheese; broccoli or spinach with olive oil and garlic
- Greek salad, and spinach pie (*spanakopita*) with rice
- Spicy bean curd with mushrooms, broccoli with black-bean sauce, vegetable fried rice, and tea
- Fresh mozzarella, basil, and tomato salad; broiled fish with vegetables and rice
- Bean burritos with rice and salad

These are examples of healthful meals you can order at most good restaurants and at Italian, Greek, Chinese, and Japanese establishments. For breakfast you can simply adapt my suggestions for what you can eat at home. Your best bets for desserts in restaurants are fresh fruit or fruit sorbet.

Once you get the idea, you can design your own meals, emphasizing the ingredients and principles that I have recommended, and adapting them to your own taste. Always remember that good food should provide pleasure and satisfaction as well as nourishment, and should support rather than undermine the body's natural healing potential.

A HEALING STORY:
A HEALTHY CIVIC LEADER

AT NINETY-THREE, Roy P. Drachman, one of the leading citizens of Tucson, Arizona, remains mentally sharp and physically active. He attributes his good health to a change of lifestyle he made forty years ago as a result of reading an article in an issue of *Forbes* magazine. The article described a man who saw his friends and contemporaries dying of heart attacks and strokes and then went to his doctor for advice and got a prescription for a healthy diet and a regular exercise. "I took the article home and gave it to my housekeeper, and I've followed the diet ever since," Roy told me.

Roy's diet emphasizes chicken, turkey, fish, and vegetables, while avoiding meat and high-fat foods. "My sin is Mexican food," he says, "but I only have it once in a while, maybe twice a month." He describes his daily routine as follows:

I arise at about 7 a.m. every day. The first thing I do is drink a large glass of water, about sixteen ounces. Then I do fifteen minutes of floor exercises prescribed for my ailing back. I have fewer aches and pains since doing them. I next take a hot shower followed by a cold shower, then shave and get dressed. I eat the same breakfast throughout the year: a large bowl of sectioned pink grapefruit and one piece of whole-wheat toast. In summer, when peaches are available, my fruit is fresh peaches with the one piece of toast. I drink no coffee or other beverage except water and a small can of grapefruit juice with Metamucil, both in the morning and in the evening just before retiring.

I usually walk two miles every day. I walk in the late afternoon in the wintertime and before breakfast on the beach in the summer months, when I'm in La Jolla, California. When I'm in Tucson, I go to the office every day, getting there no later than nine. I stay until 4:30 in the afternoon. In La Jolla I work out of my house. I have never considered retiring.

For lunch I nearly always eat a bowl of soup, sometimes with a piece of bread. About once a week, I'll have a very small piece of fruit pie, of which I eat only the fruit, or a scoop of ice cream. For dinner, I eat a very large bowl of salad—lettuce and vegetables with a small amount of dressing. The main course for dinner is a serving of vegetables, either boiled or steamed, and a very small piece of chicken, turkey, or fish (three or four ounces). I usually have a small glass of white wine before dinner. I haven't had any hard liquor for the past twenty-one years—not because it was a problem but just because I feel better without it. And I never smoked a cigarette in my life. I'm moderate in my habits. I retire about 10:30 or 11 p.m. and get about eight hours of sleep a night. I think getting the right amount of sleep is important.

Roy Drachman continues to be a civic leader who sits on many boards and is active in community affairs. As to his philosophy of life, he says, "The only religion you need is the Golden Rule. I tell my kids—your life is under your control to a great extent, including your health and your reputation. I feel the lifestyle choices I made forty years ago are responsible for my remaining healthy and active. Deciding to be conscientious about my diet was central to the change."

A HEALING STORY:
I GAVE UP FAST FOOD

SUE SOUTH grew up in the Southwest "on beans and hot dogs." She says she always ate a lot of fast food, processed foods, and prepared food. "My very favorite meals were Super Tacos and onion rings. I also had a tender spot for fried zucchini—I know there's a vegetable in there, but you kind of lose everything when it goes into the deep fryer."

Sue just turned forty and now works with the Program in Integrative Medicine in Tucson, helping to design models for training physicians in this new field. Today she eats much better food. Here is what she said when I asked her how and why she changed her diet.

Ten years ago I was diagnosed with hypogammaglobulinemia following six bouts of pneumonia in four years, four of which required hospitalization. An immunologist finally began treating me with monthly infusions of gamma globulin. Since then I've been fine except for mild asthma, which doesn't require medication. The doctor told me that I had to try to avoid people with colds, and that I had to take better care of myself, which included paying attention to my diet. He didn't give me any specific advice about diet, just told me to be careful.

At the same time I wanted to lose weight. I probably wasn't really overweight, but I thought I was. I was close to 160, but I'm tall, five feet nine inches. Anyway, I thought I'd just give up the fast food and kill two birds with one stone and probably save money too. So over the course of two days, I just stopped eating that stuff.

I didn't change the way I ate at home. I still used processed foods, and I still ate out—just not at the fast-food places.

The first thing I noticed was that I needed less sleep. I had always seemed to need ten hours a night. Within the first week of giving up fast food, I felt refreshed after just eight hours of sleep. This change has persisted. I can't say definitely that it was the result of the dietary shift, but it certainly coincided with it. I also had more energy—no question about that.

My weight started to drop. It was a gradual, healthy loss. I didn't add any exercise at that time, but I got down to where I stay now, about 140 to 145. Also, my persistent problem with constipation disappeared.

Now, as I learn more, I keep improving my diet and lifestyle. I eat chicken and turkey and very little red meat. I eat whole-grain breads and make sure I eat fruits and vegetables. All of this started with the decision to give up fast food.

I should add that I'm not religious about it. Some days I feel I just have to have a slice of pizza or a hamburger. And I do. Only now it's a special treat.

5

A MATTER OF WEIGHT

THE UNITED STATES and Canada are both experiencing an epidemic of obesity. When I return to North America from Asia or most other parts of the world, I am always amazed at how big we are, how many people in our two societies are really fat. It also seems obvious that we have been getting steadily fatter. I read recently that topping the list of Americans' gripes about everyday life is the diminishing size of seats in the coach sections of airplanes. In fact, the airlines have made coach seats a bit roomier recently, which leads me to the conclusion that passengers have gotten bigger. Recent medical evidence supports that conclusion. A survey conducted by the American Medical Association revealed that one in every five Americans was obese in 1998; in 1991 the rate was one in eight. And when I was growing up in midcentury, it was lower still.

The markets now are full of far more low-fat and nonfat foods; millions of us buy diet books and weight-loss products; millions more go to spas, weight-loss clinics, and doctors of "bariatric medicine" (specialists in obesity). And North Americans are still getting fatter than ever. Perhaps one way to understand this epidemic of obesity is to review what else has changed in our society since 1950.

An obvious possibility is that we are less active. Two inventions that contribute to inactivity are television and personal computers, both of which now draw young people into many more hours of immobility than young people experienced in the recent past. Another change is that people drive more and walk less. When I was growing up in Philadelphia, people commonly walked to neighborhood grocery stores, drugstores, and movie theaters. Today they drive to shopping malls. Urban sprawl, lack of sidewalks, and worsening air pollution in American cities all discourage walking and outdoor exercise. Less physical activity means fewer calories burned.

We are eating more now in at least two ways: We consume bigger portions and we eat more often. When I was a kid, no one got buckets of popcorn in the movies, ate oversize muffins, or drank liter-sized soft drinks. I recently bought a cookie in an airport—a popular brand that is twice as big as a cookie should be. It came in an envelope stamped with the slogan, "One Is Never Enough!" In fact, one half of a cookie this size should be plenty, but most people see these larger quantities of food as a good thing. The increased tendency to snack, eating continually from morning till night, doesn't help, and the foods we snack on—potato and corn chips, for example—are foods that promote weight gain because they are high in fat and refined carbohydrates. Fast food certainly contributes to the problem. There was very little of it at midcentury; now it is ubiquitous. Many people eat it every day and some more than once a day. This represents a change toward even greater intake of high-glycemic-index carbohydrates and fat.

Another way to get perspective on North American obesity is to look at countries where the condition is rare to try to identify differences in lifestyle. Much has been written about the French Paradox, lower-than-expected rates of coronary heart disease and heart-attack deaths in France, given the amount of fat and saturated fat consumed. This turns out to be a contentious issue, since the reporting of deaths from coronary artery disease there may not be the same as in North America, and therefore the incidence of such deaths may be higher than some of those writing about the French Paradox think. There is no argument, however, about the much lower incidence of obesity in France. You just don't see many fat French people. Yet the French not only love to eat, they love to eat butter, cream, cheese, meat, rich sauces, and rich desserts. How do they do it?

It may be that they simply don't eat as much as we do, being content with smaller portions and not indulging in all-day snacking. Another possibility is that they are more active, walking more than we do, for example. Another is that, until recently at least, they shunned fast food. Yet another is that, despite the rich desserts, they consume much less sugar than we do and less high-glycemic-index carbohydrate in general.

Japan is also a country where obesity has been extremely uncommon. Japanese love to eat and can eat a lot, but they certainly walk more than we do and consume much less fat. The fact that Japanese are beginning to get fat as they shift to Western ways of eating provides opportunities for research. One question I would love to have answered is whether rice and wheat have very different potentials to cause weight gain in people who eat them every day. Rice diets have a reputation of helping people lose weight, and the Japanese are now observing rising rates of obesity as they abandon rice for bread. Whole wheat has a higher fat content than whole rice, but I wonder if the crucial difference has to do with the form of the starch in foods prepared from these two grains. I think it is significant that rice-eating cultures eat the whole grains of that plant, even if polished, whereas wheat-eating cultures eat pulverized grains, primarily in products made from flour. If the difference turns out to be important, then overweight Westerners might do well to cut back significantly in their consumption of bread.

Losing weight has become such a cultural obsession here that people will embrace almost any scheme that promises success without asking them to give up the fattening foods they like. As I write, there are long advertisements on television for a weight-loss product called Fat Trapper. Composed mostly of chitin, the hard polysaccharide that makes up the shells of insects and crustaceans, it is supposed to bind fat in the gut and prevent its absorption. Chitin has been used to soak up oil spills, and the ads show pictures of it trapping fat in a test tube and dragging it to the bottom in a clump. But you could not eat enough chitin to make an impact on the fat you take in; if you did, it would wreak havoc with your intestinal tract and also block absorption of fat-soluble vitamins and protective phytochemicals.

The most outrageous parts of these ads, and I am sure the most effective at promoting sales, are frequent scenes of lean, attractive people helping themselves to enormous servings of high-fat foods—pizza, cheesy casseroles, cream pies, cakes—and stuffing themselves, comfortable in the knowledge that Fat Trapper is protecting them from absorbing the calories and gaining weight. And, if you order now, you get the companion product to use along with it—Exercise-in-a-Bottle—that will spare you the need of engaging in annoying physical activity. P. T. Barnum would be pleased.

The perennial success of such programs and of miracle-diet books suggests the desperation of people who are unhappy with their bodies yet cannot manage their hunger and their desire for pleasure from food. Desperate people want magical solutions: a magic formula for eating or, most of all, a magic pill that will yield the desired result without effort or sacrifice.

The pharmaceutical industry is well aware that if it could come up with such a product, it would be the best-selling drug of all time. Unfortunately, the track record of the industry in the area of weight loss is not impressive. The drugs it has brought to market either do not work or work very modestly; those that work best are toxic, causing such problems as addiction, cataracts, and heart damage. The current offering, orlistat (Xenical), promises minimal weight loss in long-term usage when combined with calorie restriction and exercise—not exactly the magic pill we've been waiting for—and can interfere with intestinal function.

Still, there are those who hope that ongoing research on hormonal regulation of metabolism may uncover possibilities for pharmacological intervention. Great fanfare a few years ago accompanied the discovery of leptin, a hormone that controls satiety, but to date nothing of practical value in the treatment and prevention of obesity has come of it. A basic problem is that interference in the mechanics of energy production and use in the human body is likely to have unforeseen, serious adverse effects. I would advise great caution in trying any new pharmaceutical drugs for weight loss until they have been around long enough to make doctors confident of their safety and efficacy.

Unfortunately, the basic equation that relates caloric intake to weight is very simple. If caloric intake consistently exceeds caloric expenditure, the body will tend to store excess calories as fat. The simple fact is that so many Americans are fat because they are eating far more calories than they expend in their activities of daily living, and many people are simply unconscious of the excess calories they eat. Nutritionists recommend that moderately active adults consume between 2,000 and 3,000 calories a day, depending on gender and body size. If you are not careful about your food choices and portions, you can easily pack away 1,500 calories or more at breakfast, then have two more meals that will put you way over the top, not counting snacks.

Recently, I picked up the food section of the morning newspaper in Tucson, Arizona, and read the results of a recipe contest for best potluck entrée. Here is one of the winning entries:

✍ *Green Chile Macaroni and Cheese* ✍

1 pound dry pasta, preferably penne
2 quarts heavy cream
¼ cup yellow onion, chopped
6 cloves garlic, chopped
1 cup fresh mild green chile, chopped
1 tablespoon olive oil
1 pound sharp cheddar cheese, shredded
½ pound mozzarella cheese, shredded
salt and pepper to taste
½ cup cilantro, coarsely chopped

I'm not going to reprint the directions that follow, because I don't want you even to think about making this dish, even as an occasional indulgence. The recipe says it yields six servings, each providing 1,803 calories, 150 grams of fat (accounting for 73 percent of the calories), 46 grams of protein, 71 grams of carbohydrate, and 535 milligrams of cholesterol. In other words, one serving of this main dish gives you virtually all of your caloric requirement for the day. If this is mainstream food, then I repeat my assertion that the reason so many Americans are fat is simply that they eat too much and too much of the wrong things.

It is true, however, that certain factors can influence the basic equation.

First and foremost is genetics. I have already mentioned the existence of so-called thrifty genes that allow some people to store up available calories as fat more readily than others. Such genes were a great advantage in populations that often lived near starvation or went through periodic cycles of feast and famine. Our distant hominid ancestors probably lived mostly in those conditions, which would have selected for the genes in question. And probably that is why so many people today have that genetic constitution. A common complaint of the overweight is: I can gain weight just by looking at food. They have to do more than look at it, of course, but it is quite true that many of us are genetically programmed to turn available calories into fat as efficiently as possible. The problem is that those genes are no longer advantageous, with food and calories now always available to us in abundance and excess. All of us also know people who eat constantly and remain lean. In fact, some of them want to gain weight and complain of an inability to do so. They have a different sort of genetic constitution and metabolism (and would not fare well if the food supply failed).

The principal mechanism by which genes regulate hunger and body fat is through an appetite control center in the hypothalamus, a deep brain structure that regulates many body functions. In each of us, this mechanism is set to a certain point, mostly determined by genes and relatively resistant to change. The setting keeps us at a certain weight, compensating for changes in activity and variations in caloric intake. This is the main reason that dieting is so frustrating. As you reduce caloric intake, the hypothalamus alters metabolism to increase the efficiency of turning calories into stored fat. And because a reducing diet, by definition, is a temporary regimen, as soon as you go off it, you will regain the weight.

The only ways I know to alter the hypothalamic set point for appetite are exercise and stimulant drugs. In addition to increasing caloric output, regular exercise—an increase in daily physical activity, not Exercise-in-a-Bottle—can, over time, change the basic equation in your favor and help you lose weight and keep it off. Similarly, stimulant drugs like amphetamine, cocaine, ephedrine, caffeine, nicotine, and phenylpropanolamine (PPA) promote weight loss by an effect on the hypothalamic hunger center. Unfortunately, they are addictive, have potentially harmful physical and psychological side effects, lose their effectiveness over time, and set you up for rebound weight gain as soon as you discontinue them. (Some are also illegal.)

So the standard, sensible advice from nutritionists and physicians to people who want to lose weight has been and still is the following:

- take account of the basic equation and do not fall for fad diets or weight-loss scams
- cut caloric intake by cutting calories while maintaining the recommended proportions of carbohydrate, fat, and protein in the diet
- increase caloric output by increasing physical activity

There may be other possibilities, but before I mention them, I must address the cultural issues surrounding obesity. Being fat is a major disadvantage in our society, because it puts you at odds with prevailing standards of beauty and sexual attractiveness. I wrote earlier that some cultures—Polynesians and gypsies, for two—do not share those standards. Nor have they been in force throughout Western history. Not too long ago, stout men and buxom women were in fashion and desirable. I find it interesting that in cultures that like body fat and see it as beautiful there is little concern about it being unhealthful. In fact, people in those cultures equate ample girth not only with prosperity but also with health of body, mind, and spirit.

In our culture, there is a great deal of medical rationalization to justify our dislike of fat. Doctors and public health experts tell us constantly about the hazards of carrying too much weight around: increased risks of cardiovascular disease, diabetes, certain cancers, and joint problems to name a few. Now, there is obesity and there is obesity. We all know morbid obesity when we see it, and can easily understand how it increases the workload of the heart and lungs, interferes with physical movement, and takes a heavy emotional toll. But the majority of people obsessed with losing weight are not in this category, even if the amount of fat on their bodies is more than the culture deems appropriate and much more than they would like to have. I am not convinced that those people are necessarily compromising their health by weighing more than tables of ideal weight say they should, especially if they are keeping fit and otherwise taking good care of themselves.

The fact is that Western medicine, being part of Western culture, has taken on its prejudice against body fat. That attitude, I believe, has warped medical research and practice, compromising objectivity in assessing the actual health hazards of obesity. For example, most doctors assume that being fat decreases longevity, and that losing weight will increase it, but recent studies by exercise physiologists cast doubt on that assumption. If fat people remain active and head off further weight gains, there is no association between being fat and dying early.

So if you are not morbidly obese and you are willing to be active, to keep yourself fit, and maintain a healthy lifestyle in other ways, you may be able to ignore the pronouncements of doctors and rest assured that you will live as long and as healthy a life as people like you who are lean. Then why worry about losing weight? The answer, probably, is that you do not like yourself the way you are, the way nature, genes, and your hypothalamus want to keep you. If that's the case, I would ask you to consider, at least, the possibility of working on that attitude, of practicing self-acceptance, and trying to like your body the way nature designed it. Remind yourself that fashions in bodies, like fashions in clothes, are arbitrary; they come and go. You could have been born in a time and place where leanness was out of fashion and thin people were considered unattractive and unhealthy. I realize that most of you overweight readers are not going to accept that, but I still want you to think about it.

But let's say you really do want to get your weight down. How can you use the information I have given you about nutrition and the optimum diet to do so?

First of all, you have to pay attention to the basic equation and both cut caloric intake and increase caloric expenditure. I agree with nutritionists who say that cutting caloric intake means cutting calories across the board, rather than making any drastic changes in the ideal proportions of macronutrients. You should continue to eat about 50 to 60 percent of calories as carbohydrate, 30 percent as fat, and 10 to 20 percent as protein, but you must reduce the amount you eat, both by decreasing the size of portions and by cutting down on snacking, especially the kind of unconscious snacking that many people do as a nervous habit.

That does not mean eating three meager meals a day. If you approach weight loss with a mind-set of deprivation, you will not succeed. Instead you must find a way to eat less while managing your hunger. Hunger management is not just about taking care of physical appetite. It also includes satisfying the desire for pleasure from food in all of its aspects. If you don't satisfy hunger during the day, you may find yourself eating everything in sight in the evening until you have taken in more calories than if you were not trying to reduce your intake. I notice that if I get nothing but terrible food—say, during a long day of travel that condemns me to airport and airline meals—my craving for good food gets really strong even if I've eaten enough calories for the day's activity.

For me, hunger management means making sure I eat good food regularly. For others, it might mean eating frequently—five or six smaller meals throughout the day rather than the traditional three.

Everyone is different, and everyone trying to reduce caloric intake needs to satisfy their hunger in one way or another. If you find you simply cannot eat less, you may need to consult a nutritionist or dietitian for help with hunger management.

There are also some practical strategies to try. The sight of food in variety and abundance stimulates overeating, which is why buffet dining can be disastrous. Try to avoid tempting displays of food. Try not to shop for food when you are hungry. Experiment with removing platters of food after you have served yourself; better they should be out of sight in the kitchen than in view on the table. If possible, do not spend time in the company of persons who overeat or who encourage you to overeat.

Although I have stated my objections to low-carbohydrate diets, I think the relationship between carbohydrate and obesity deserves more attention. Walter Willett, the champion of the Mediterranean diet, believes that refined carbohydrate—flour and sugar, especially— is the chief culprit in the Western diet responsible for obesity. I agree with him and recommend that people trying to lose weight reduce intake of these foods, using more whole-grain products and fruit.

Also, I am impressed by the number of people who go on low-carbohydrate diets and report that cravings for carbohydrates— sweets, especially—disappear, even as they lose weight. These are probably carbohydrate-sensitive individuals who do especially poorly with high-glycemic loads of refined starch and sugar. They should be able to eat modest amounts of low-glycemic-index foods like whole grains, firm-cooked pasta, and fruits like berries and cherries. Some people tell me they have lost weight just by cutting out bread. I wrote earlier that most bread today has a very high glycemic index, because of the nature of the flour used to make it. I can believe that if you have thrifty genes and so gain weight easily, being careful about the amount and kind of carbohydrate foods you eat is the single best strategy you can use to control your weight. A good place to start is by cutting way down on foods made with sugar and flour.

That does not mean following the Atkins diet or one of its spin-offs. Those diets appeal mostly to people who love meat and fat, who can do without starch and sugar, and never liked vegetables much anyway. The central problem with them is that they provide much too much protein (the consequences of which on liver and kidney function may not show up until much later in life), too much saturated fat, and, far from least important, too few of the protective factors in fruits and vegetables that are your best protection against cancer and the degenerative diseases of later life. For short-term weight loss, they are probably all right—as good as any other crash diet—but as a long-term eating strategy, they expose the body to harmful elements in food and leave it unprotected.

Perhaps unwise choices of carbohydrates explain why North Americans have grown fatter even as they have had more low-fat and nonfat food options to help them control their weight. Look at the explosion of popularity of nonfat frozen yogurt, now a favorite snack food, served up at airports, in cafeterias, and almost everywhere. Nonfat frozen yogurt is full of sugar, but people think of it as a dietetic alternative to ice cream. Many who used to indulge in ice cream once a week might now have frozen yogurt every day. I know people who gobble fat-free cookies by the handful, as if they were calorie-free or even had "negative calories." In fact, these very popular foods of recent invention are high in refined carbohydrate calories and add to the glycemic load that pushes carbohydrate-sensitive individuals toward further storage of caloric energy as body fat.

You should also note that the epidemic of obesity here also correlates with widespread use of noncaloric artificial sweeteners and, more recently, with the noncaloric fat substitute olestra. Artificial sweeteners may be useful for diabetics, but there is no evidence that they help anyone lose weight—not surprising, since people usually add them to items in meals already top-heavy in calories and refined carbohydrates. And I consider all of them suspect in terms of long-range effects on health.

As for olestra, a nonabsorbable molecule that has the mouth feel and cooking properties of fat, it is now used to create fat-free potato chips, corn chips, and other snack foods and may soon be approved for many more products, including cookies and cakes. Consumer advocates have attacked it for blocking absorption of fat-soluble vitamins (which can be added to foods as supplements to compensate for any losses) and causing intestinal upheavals in some people, but the real problem is elsewhere. The use of this fake fat simply encourages greater consumption of low-quality, refined-carbohydrate foods that are often high in sodium, full of unhealthful additives, and devoid of protective nutritional factors. People who eat them, probably more frequently and in greater quantity than they would eat the original versions, will be increasing their tendency to gain weight by taking in more of the wrong kind of calories.

I should mention one other possible influence on the basic equation that comes from my own experience and that of people I know, but for which there is no scientific evidence from research studies. I have found that at certain times in my life, my metabolism has shifted for periods of a few days to a few weeks in the direction that I wish it would stay—where my weight is steady or even drops without effort no matter how I eat. During these periods I feel energized, creative, and quite happy with, and accepting of, my body. I wish I knew what goes on at these times. Is the metabolic change a result of a particular state of mind? Do these periods represent an alteration of the hypo-thalamic set point in response to altered genetic instructions? If so, what event, internal or external, might trigger the change? I know only that one's state of consciousness can affect physiology, and I think it is worth paying attention to correlations between your mind and your metabolism. If you can identify a particular mental/emotional state with enhanced metabolism, you can practice staying in that state more of the time.

A number of weight-conscious friends, colleagues, and patients have told me stories of vacationing in such countries as France and Italy, eating everything they wanted for several weeks with no thought of the consequences, then returning home to face the scales and discovering to their astonishment and delight that they had gained not at all or even lost a bit. Some of them insist they had no increase of physical activity during these times and cannot explain what happened. They wonder if the quality of food in the countries they visited was different or if their attitude about eating good food without anxiety was responsible. Again, I'm afraid I have no answers for them but would love to know.

Finally, I want to say a few words about fasting. Abstaining from food has significant effects on body and mind. It can make more energy available to the body, at least temporarily, because digestion requires energy. For this reason, fasting at the onset of a cold can shorten its duration. Fasting can also be a technique to sharpen con-centration, help you gain insight into the nature of the mind, and even develop spiritual awareness (hence its association with religious observances). It is not, however, a way to lose weight. Fasting prepares the body for starvation, slowing metabolism and promoting storage of calories as fat when eating resumes.

Now a summary of what I have been telling you about weight:

- The basic equation relating calories in to calories out rules. If you consistently eat more calories than you burn, you will tend to store up the excess as body fat.
- Your weight and tendency to gain weight are strongly determined by your genes and mediated through regulation of the hypothalamic hunger center in the brain.
- Many people are genetically programmed to put weight on whenever calories are available in abundance in the body.
- Exercise and stimulant drugs can change the set point of the hypothalamic hunger center in the direction favoring weight loss (though stimulants should be avoided). Possibly, certain states of consciousness can also do it.
- Ordinary obesity should be distinguished from morbid obesity, which seriously interferes with health and movement and is a medical concern.
- Strong cultural prejudice against ample body fat in our societies has influenced Western medical research, teaching, and practice, compromising their objectivity in assessing the health consequences of being fatter than the ideal body weights of standardized tables.
- If you weigh more than you "should" but are not morbidly obese, you must try to remain physically fit and active and commit to living a healthful lifestyle in order to minimize the chance that being heavy will shorten your life or increase your risks of chronic disease.
- If your only reason for wanting to lose weight is unhappiness with your body, try to work on changing your attitude toward your body in addition to anything you do to try to lose weight.
- Avoid *all* diet products, including supplements, foods, herbs, potions, and books (not to mention doctors, drugs, clinics, and programs) that promise weight loss without changing what you eat or the size of your portions.
- Avoid diets that call for radical reshuffling of proportions of macronutrients, such as very low fat and very low carbohydrate diets, as long-term eating plans.

- To lose weight, decrease caloric intake across the board, maintaining the recommended proportions of macronutrients: 50 to 60 percent of calories from carbohydrate, 30 percent from fat, and 10 to 20 percent from protein.
- Pay careful attention to the amount and kind of carbohydrate calories you ingest, minimizing intake of refined starch and sugar and high-glycemic-index foods. In particular, minimize consumption of common forms of bread and other foods made from wheat flour.
- Be wary of low-fat and nonfat snacks and sweets that are high in refined carbohydrates.
- Avoid artificial sweeteners and products made with them or with the fat substitute olestra.
- Be wary of new pharmaceutical treatments for weight loss until medical consensus declares them to be safe and effective.
- Increase caloric expenditure by increasing physical activity. The kind of activity that may be most effective at promoting weight loss may be general activity throughout the day, rather than intense, isolated workouts. Walking, climbing stairs, housework, gardening all contribute. Try to move more.
- Dieting is not the answer to keeping weight down. As you have heard many times, almost all people who diet to lose weight regain it (and more). Instead, you need to change long-term patterns of eating and physical activity. Hunger management is key. New patterns of eating must satisfy both physical hunger and the need for sensory pleasure from food.
- Estimate your average daily caloric intake by adding up the calories you eat each day for a week. (Use standard tables of food composition to do so. And consult the breakdowns on packages of food you consume.) Remember, it is very easy to run up total calories way above daily needs. Once you have determined your average daily caloric intake, it is not necessary to count calories all the time. Just try to keep in mind how much food you really need, given your level of physical activity.
- Pay particular attention to portion size of foods you like to eat. Develop a sense of appropriate portions, by reading labels, measuring, and weighing foods.
- Avoid buffets and situations in which you are tempted by large servings of food. Keep serving platters out of sight whenever possible.

- If you like to snack, learn to snack on less-calorie-dense foods and pay attention to the amounts you eat. If you have to have some chips, go for brands made with less fat and the right kind of fat, and eat a handful rather than the whole bag. Try snacking on fruit, raw vegetables, some nuts, even a piece of dark chocolate if you crave a sweet.
- Finally, if you are going to eat too much, as you sometimes will, remember that it is better to eat too much good food than too much bad food.

The remainder of this book is about buying and preparing delicious, healthful food—the kind of food that, eaten sensibly and included in an active lifestyle, can help you maintain the weight that works best for you.

A HEALING STORY: CONQUERING AN EATING DISORDER

DEBRA DUBOIS is forty-four and is one of my assistants. I was surprised when she told me she had had an eating disorder, because she seemed to eat mostly good food in moderation. This is what she told me:

I grew up on a farm in Iowa and moved to Arizona in the sixth grade, where I was the fattest kid in the class. None of my three sisters was heavy. I had always been told to clean my plate and ate a lot of meat, soda, and sugar as a kid. As I got older, my self-esteem really suffered because of my weight. I tried diet pills, legal and illegal. They worked but put me all over the place emotionally. At age nineteen, after the birth of my oldest daughter, I ballooned up to 185 pounds.

At that point I started to binge and purge. I got the idea from the media. I kept my behavior secret. As a result of that, and by no longer drinking soda, I lost fifty pounds by the time my second child came. I was experiencing physical and sexual abuse in my marriage. Eating and purging gave me a sense of control over at least one area of my life.

When I was about twenty-four, I started my own garden, gave up meat, and began eating whole grains. I also stopped using diet pills, replacing them with coffee—a lot of coffee, at least one pot a day.

About three years ago, I finally got past the bulimia. I had to learn to love myself, end bad relationships, and look at food differently. I did all this by myself; I never sought or got any professional help.

Looking back on it, I'm amazed. I was married fourteen years, and my husband never knew I was bulimic. I threw up after most meals and at business meetings. I could do it very quickly and secretively. (I had certain trigger foods like pizza and ice cream, which I could vomit easily.) I definitely damaged my body. My esophagus is scarred, and my dental enamel is gone.

Now I look at meals as a ritual. I always eat breakfast and always make myself sit down to dinner, even if I'm by myself. I cook a lot and like to experiment in the kitchen. And I really enjoy food, all the flavors and textures. I like to try out different seasonings and always travel with a bottle of Tabasco sauce. I don't deprive myself of anything, even pizza and ice cream. I think if you deprive yourself, you want it more. I don't like to eat after 6 p.m.—my body says no.

I've replaced all the coffee with some green tea, which works well for me. It seems to have mellowed me out. And the allergic rhinitis and bronchitis I always had have lessened since I began drinking it.

My younger kids, nine and eleven, are good eaters. My older son is a vegetarian. My oldest daughter is obese, but none of the children have had eating disorders.

My weight now shifts between 135 and 140 pounds, but it's stable in that range. If I feel like I'm gaining weight, I'll do a juice fast for a day and eat lots of sushi. I hike for exercise. I think when I was bulimic I was always on the run. Food wasn't the enemy—it was my own demons. I think I have a good relationship with food now. Unless you sit down and take time to enjoy what you're eating, you can't really appreciate it.

6

BUYING FOOD
AND EATING OUT
(WITH A WORD ABOUT VIBRATIONS)

A DISH can only be as good as its worst ingredient. The optimum diet begins with knowledge of how to buy food, both for home preparation and for when you are eating away from home.

I find that when I go to a supermarket, I make most of my purchases from the periphery of the store, especially the produce section, and few from the interior, which is mostly full of processed, packaged, canned, and frozen foods. I shop frequently at natural food stores, especially the newer natural food supermarkets that I hope will become the grocery stores of tomorrow. In addition to a wider range of fruits and vegetables, including much organic produce, they carry all the soy foods, drug- and hormone-free meats and poultry, good prepared foods, and a full line of dietary supplements. I also belong to a buying club that places a monthly order with a local natural foods cooperative that offers near-wholesale prices on organic grains, nuts, flours, seeds, oils, and many other products I use frequently.

The most important piece of advice I can give you about shopping for food is to read labels. The information on food labels is now more complete and easier to read than ever. Begin by reading the list of ingredients, which are in descending order, from those present in the greatest amount to those present in the least. I usually reject any product whose list of ingredients is too long, the print too fine, and the space on the label barely adequate to contain it. I always look for the words partially hydrogenated—a cause for automatic rejection. And there are many food additives I won't eat, which I will discuss shortly.

Then I look at the information under Nutrition Facts, starting with calories per serving and the breakdown into macronutrients. You should note the percentage of fat calories and the relative contribution of saturated, monounsaturated, and polyunsaturated fat. Also note cholesterol and sodium content. Check the total of carbohydrates and the amount of sugar and fiber, if any. Also look for the presence of vitamins and key minerals like iron and calcium.

Let me show you how to be a good label detective by reviewing with you the information on several representative products: some good, some bad, some ugly. I'll start with a carton of organic vegetable broth from the new natural foods section of a local supermarket. The label boasts that the broth is "all natural" and "fat-free," with "no MSG added." (MSG, monosodium glutamate, is a flavor enhancer, and one of the additives I would rather not eat.) The ingredients in this product are: "filtered water, organic carrots, organic celery, organic onion, organic leeks, organic tomato, organic garlic, sea salt, bay leaves, parsley, thyme," and the label further states that the vegetables were grown and processed in accordance with organic agriculture codes in Oregon and California. This looks great— nothing in it I would not use myself in making a vegetable broth at home. I would, however, prefer a salt-free version so that I could season it myself, especially since a one-cup serving has 670 milligrams of sodium, almost a third of the recommended daily intake (which some experts would say is already too high).

The Nutrition Facts portion of the label, where I found the sodium content, confirms that the broth is fat-free and, in fact, mostly calorie-free. It provides tiny amounts (2 and 6 percent respectively) of the daily recommended quantities of calcium and iron. So, all in all, it is a good product, useful as a soup base, convenient as a flavorful addition to the liquid for cooking grains and vegetables. When using it, you would just want to taste dishes carefully to avoid oversalting them.

Next, from the same part of the store, I have a natural soup-in-a-cup, "Pasta Parmesan," ready almost instantly with the addition of boiling water. The label says it's fat- and cholesterol-free with

"40% less sodium than other leading brands." The list of ingredients looks rather long, but when I read it, I am reassured; the manufacturer has been conscientious in spelling everything out. It reads: "Linguine pasta (100% semolina flour), dehydrated vegetables (tomatoes, onions, peas, carrots, broccoli, red bell peppers, garlic), soy granules, soy sauce powder (soybeans, wheat, salt), natural flavors (no MSG), yeast extract, vinegar powder, Parmesan cheese (milk, cheese culture, salt, enzymes), sea salt, parsley, oregano, rosemary, white pepper, cayenne pepper, thyme, bay leaves, potato flour, natural beta carotene." This is all familiar stuff—nothing bad. The vegetables listed are not organic, but the amounts of them are so small as to make that insignificant.

The Nutrition Facts look good, too: 100 calories per serving, no fat or cholesterol, only 290 milligrams of sodium, most of the calories (80) from carbohydrate and the rest (20) from protein, and a bit of beta-carotene and vitamin C. But wait! I assumed the product contained one serving, but on closer inspection I read, "Servings per container: about 2." I consider this deceptive. Maybe a small child would be happy with this as a serving, but all adults I know would eat the whole thing. That means 200 calories, not 100, and almost 600 milligrams of sodium, almost as much as in our salty broth above. If this truly represents "40% less sodium than other leading brands," just imagine how much excess sodium people get from eating leading brands.

Let's try a healthy cracker, a form of Swedish crispbread from a regular supermarket. The package says it's all natural, fat- and cholesterol-free, and made with "100% whole grain rye." The U.S.D.A. Food Guide Pyramid is reproduced in color here, with its base of "bread, cereal, rice, and pasta" highlighted, and the list of ingredients is satisfyingly short: "Whole grain rye flour, yeast, salt." One cracker, we learn, has 45 calories, most from carbohydrate and a little from protein, along with two grams of fiber. Two of these would give you a tenth of your daily fiber requirement, not as much as you might expect given their rough appearance. Sodium is only 40 milligrams per cracker, pretty good. This product is fine.

Finally, let's look at a can of fat-free, vegetarian baked beans, also from a regular supermarket. The writing on the label tells us it's "high in fiber." The ingredients are "prepared white beans, water, brown sugar, sugar, tomato paste, salt, corn starch, mustard, onion powder, spices, extractive of paprika, garlic powder, and natural flavor." The Nutrition Facts label tells us that a serving size is one-half cup, but, again, I would be more likely to eat a cup. One cup of these beans has 260 calories, 192 from carbohydrate (including 32 from sugar, not so much) and the rest from protein. It also provides a very respectable 12 grams of fiber—almost a third of the recommended daily intake—along with some vitamin A, iron, and calcium. The only bad news is high sodium —1,100 milligrams—as we have seen, a common problem with prepared foods and of concern mainly to the salt-sensitive.

These are examples of relatively healthful products available now in regular grocery stores. All of them get high marks for being free of bad ingredients and additives.

For the next batch of products I ventured into the interior depths of the supermarket, going to sections I rarely visit. I came out first with a package of flour tortillas, sporting label banners reading "Premium Quality" and "No Lard, No Cholesterol." Here are the ingredients: "Enriched, bleached flour (flour, niacin, iron, thiamin mononitrate, riboflavin, folic acid), water, vegetable shortening (partially hydrogenated soybean and/or cottonseed oils), contains 2% or less of the following: salt, leavening (baking soda, sodium aluminum sulfate, cornstarch, monocalcium phosphate, and/or sodium acid pyrophosphate, calcium sulfate), propionic acid, calcium propionate, sorbic acid, potassium sorbate, benzoic acid, and phosphoric acid (to preserve freshness), dough conditioners (fumaric acid, L-cysteine, sodium metabisulfite)."

That seems like a lot of unfamiliar stuff, but, actually, the worst ingredients are right at the beginning: enriched, bleached flour—the prototypical refined carbohydrate—and vegetable shortening, which immediately disqualifies the product for inclusion in the optimum diet. The chemical ingredients are mostly innocuous: B vitamins, leavening agents, and preservatives to retard mold growth. I would prefer not to eat the preservatives, but I would less like to eat a moldy flour tortilla.

One tortilla (weighing 51 grams) has 160 calories, 40 of them from fat and 10 of those from saturated fat; 360 milligrams of sodium; and only 1 gram of fiber. Most of the calories come from high-glycemic-index carbohydrate. This product goes back on the shelf. (I can order from my natural foods cooperative a brand of whole-wheat flour tortillas, made with organic wheat and no added fat.)

Next I've got a bag of something called "Cheesy ZigZags," "cheese-flavored snacks" that brag they are "dangerously cheesy." Here we go: "Enriched corn meal (corn meal, ferrous sulfate, niacin, thiamin mononitrate, riboflavin, and folic acid), vegetable oil contains one or more of the following: corn, cottonseed, partially hydrogenated [cottonseed or soybean] or hydrogenated [corn or cottonseed] oil), whey, salt, cheddar cheese (cultured milk, salt, enzymes), maltodextrin, disodium phosphate, sour cream (cultured cream, nonfat milk), artificial flavor, monosodium glutamate, lactic acid, artificial colors (yellow 6, extractives of turmeric and annatto), and citric acid."

In addition to the problems of refined carbohydrate—this time in the form of finely milled corn meal—and the terrible fat, we have monosodium glutamate and yellow 6, a synthetic food dye. Here is what my source book on food additives says of this dye:

FD&C [food, drug & cosmetic] Yellow No. 6 (Sunset Yellow)— This has been shown to cause allergic reactions like hives, rhinitis (runny nose), and nasal congestion. It appeared to cause tumors of the kidney and adrenal glands in rats, and it may be carcinogenic. FDA reviewed studies on rats and believes that this color is safe to use. This color is banned in Norway and Sweden. It has been found used in sausages, candy, gelatin, and baked goods.

The real shock comes under Nutrition Facts. The bag contains 10 ounces (283.5 grams) of bright-orange ZigZags and says this is ten servings. I think most people would eat a quarter of the bag at once. If you did, you would consume 425 calories, of which 250, or 59 percent, would be fat. That snack might give you nearly a quarter of your total caloric requirement for the day and almost half of the fat calories you need. Needless to say, it would not be good fat. The fiber you would get from this would be about 2 grams—next to nothing—and the sodium a hefty 925 milligrams. Back on the shelf with it.

The next item is a box of "sweetened rice cereal" just for kids, made by one of the major cereal manufacturers. It has a kid-friendly name, and the box is decorated with currently popular cartoon characters and bright colors designed to make your children nag you to buy it for them. The cereal consists of purple flakes mixed with green reptile-shaped bits (!). The label identifies the product as a "low fat, cholesterol-free food" with "10 essential vitamins and minerals." Here come the ingredients: "Sugar, rice, rice flour, hydrogenated vegetable oil (coconut and palm kernel oils), corn syrup, salt, malted barley and corn extract, malted barley flour, wheat starch, yellow 5, red 40, blue 1, blue 2." There follows a separate listing of the added vitamins (A, Bs, and D) and minerals (iron and zinc).

Note that the first ingredient is sugar, even ahead of the grains, a good example of the problem of added sugar in processed foods. All grains in this mix are refined. The fat is highly saturated, and there is a rainbow of chemical dyes. My source book says to use yellow 5 (tartrazine) with caution because it may cause allergic reactions and, in children, behavioral problems (worsening of hyperactivity and attention-deficit disorder). It also advises caution about red 40, one of the newer food dyes developed to replace other, banned reds. Red 40 is suspected of being carcinogenic. "It is the most widely used food color and is mainly used in junk foods," according to my reference guide. The book has stronger warnings about the two blues, which it says should be avoided:

FD&C Blue No. 1 (Brilliant Blue)—It is found in desserts, confectioneries, candies, and beverages. It has not been properly tested and [is] suspected to contain a small cancer risk. It is banned in Finland and France.

FD&C Blue No. 2 (Indigotine/Indigo-carmine)—Not much is known of this additive, although it was suspected to cause brain tumors in animals. It can cause allergic reactions. Aside from soft drinks, candy, and baked products, it is also found in pet foods. This is banned in Norway.

This cereal is, indeed, low fat, with only 10 percent of its calories from fat, but all of that is saturated. The carbohydrate content is dreadful. I hope you can resist your children's clamoring for cutely packaged foods that are loaded with unhealthful ingredients.

Finally, let's have dessert. How about "Real Cheesecake" mix, a no-bake dessert from one of the biggest manufacturers of processed food? If I were going to make a cheesecake at home, the only ingredients I would use would be cream cheese, sour cream, eggs, sugar, vanilla, lemon juice, and a crumb crust of pulverized Graham crackers, butter, and sugar. (I don't make cheesecakes at home; they have too much saturated fat and too much dairy protein for me.) Here are the ingredients of this mix: "**Filling:** sugar, baker's cheese (skim milk, lactic acid, cultures), hydrogenated coconut oil, corn syrup, modified food starch, sodium phosphate (for thickening), partially hydrogenated palm kernel oil, sodium caseinate (from milk), propylene glycol monostearate (for blending), dipotassium phosphate, salt, mono- and diglycerides (for blending), whey (from milk), hydroxylated soy lecithin and acetylated monoglycerides (for blending), BHA (preservative), yellow 5, artificial flavor, natural flavor, yellow 6, beta carotene (color), citric acid (preservative). **Crust:** enriched wheat flour (flour, niacin, reduced iron, thiamin mononitrate, riboflavin, folic acid), Graham flour, sugar, partially hydrogenated vegetable oil (soybean and/or cottonseed and/or canola oils), molasses, high fructose corn syrup, salt, baking soda, BHA, TBHQ, and citric acid (preservatives)."

I don't think that needs any comment, and after copying it down, I have such a headache that I can't even bear to look at the Nutrition Facts.

I hope I have given you some sense of the importance of reading labels on food products you are thinking of buying. Let me summarize for you some of my advice about them:

- Try to buy foods that contain the same ingredients you would use at home.
- Avoid products that have so many ingredients they barely fit on the label.
- Watch for bad ingredients like partially hydrogenated oils.
- Avoid products containing artificial colors, artificial sweeteners, nitrites or nitrates, sulfites, potassium bromate, and brominated vegetable oil. In my opinion, all of these pose health risks.
- Minimize consumption of products containing MSG (monosodium glutamate), aluminum, and the preservatives BHA, BHT, and TBHQ. In my opinion, these may pose health risks.
- In checking Nutrition Facts on food labels, make sure the serving size is what you would actually eat, and adjust the arithmetic accordingly.

When you are eating out, you obviously cannot read the labels of the products used in a restaurant and you cannot know how carefully a restaurant manager shops, but you can improve your chances of getting high-quality food by making wise choices about where to eat and what to order. I enjoy good restaurants, and in them I like eating dishes I am unlikely to make at home. When I travel, I have to eat out, though not always where I'd like to. But I have found it easier in recent years to get healthful food in restaurants. Many now offer low-fat, vegetarian, and heart-healthful main dishes; many have fresh fish; and some even emphasize organic produce and animal foods. I know I can always get a healthful meal of sushi (and *edamame*) at better Japanese restaurants, vegetarian appetizers made with olive oil at Middle Eastern and Greek restaurants, pasta with marinara sauce and a good salad at Italian restaurants, and stir-fried vegetables and tofu at Chinese ones. Often I eat fish when I eat out, because the quality of fish available at good restaurants is usually better than what I can get to cook at home.

I am sure I do not have to tell you that there are many pitfalls to restaurant dining. Here are some tips for avoiding them:

- Portions of food in restaurants are often much too large. Don't always finish everything you are served. Consider splitting dishes with fellow diners, taking the excess home, or just leaving it on the plate. A friend of mine was once dining at a fashionable restaurant with the comedian George Burns and asked him how he stayed so thin when he ate out so often. Burns looked up and growled, "Eat half!"
- Avoid buffets. The sight of large quantities of food, attractively presented, encourages overeating.
- Don't automatically eat bread and butter while waiting for your first course. Most restaurant bread is of the fluffy, white, high-glycemic-index sort, and you can take in far too many calories with it before you even get to an appetizer. If you find it hard to resist, ask the waiter not to bring bread until the rest of the food is ready. Eat small amounts, and if you have to have fat with it, ask for extra-virgin olive oil. Many restaurants now offer it as an alternative to butter.
- Ask for salad dressing on the side, so that you can put the amount

on you want. Choose olive-oil vinaigrettes if available. Or simply ask for olive oil, vinegar, and lemon if you wish.

- Avoid cream-based soups.
- Also ask for sauces on the side, since they are usually high in saturated fat.
- Avoid fried foods.
- Ask for grilled or broiled fish to be prepared without butter.
- Ask for vegetables that are steamed or prepared with olive oil instead of butter.
- If you order rich desserts, try to satisfy yourself with a few bites rather than eating the whole thing.
- If the water you are served tastes like chlorine, order bottled water.

I also want to discuss a topic I consider important that nutritionists, dietitians, and doctors never mention: the spiritual quality of food. People in many cultures believe that food conveys something more than the sum of its nutrients—a form of vital energy that we need or even the emotional and spiritual vibrations of people who have handled it. I share those beliefs, but I want to make clear that I have no scientific evidence to support them and consider this whole aspect of food to exist in a realm separate from that studied by the sciences of biochemistry and nutrition.

Obviously, there are differences between limp, tired carrots with yellow-green tops lying on the dry shelf of a convenience store and spiffy, bright-orange-and-green carrots nestling under a mister in a natural foods supermarket. Some of those differences have objective correlates. Under a microscope, for example, we might see protoplasm in the cells of the better-looking carrots streaming more briskly than in cells of the tired ones. It would be fair to say that the latter had more vital energy than the former, a distinction that might have to do with dehydration, length of time since harvesting, temperature, and so forth, all of which are measurable. The better-looking carrots will certainly be crunchier and might taste better, too. If both had the same content of macronutrients and micronutrients, would there be a difference in nutritional value apart from any difference in taste or aesthetic appeal? I suspect so.

What if we were to compare bunches of organically grown and

conventionally grown carrots of equal freshness? Some organic carrots I have tasted have been deliciously sweet, much more flavorful than their conventional counterparts. Apparently, they had a higher sugar content. Was this due to varietal, that is, genetic, differences or to the growing methods—nature or nurture? A bit of existing research suggests that organically grown fruits and vegetables have higher nutritional content than conventional forms. I would like to see agricultural scientists investigate this subject vigorously.

Now, suppose we ask two different people to make soup from the same batch of carrots. The first cook is angry and resentful of the assignment but follows our recipe exactly. The second is centered and peaceful and prepares the same recipe with love and a desire to give enjoyment to those who will eat it. Is there any difference between the two batches of soup? Would people eating them have different experiences or receive different influences on their bodies, minds, or spirits? I doubt that we could document such differences with our present methods. Controlled trials will probably not settle the question. Nevertheless, I believe there are differences.

Most of us intuitively accept the possibility that food prepared with love is better for us than food prepared without it. The comfort provided by a bowl of mother's soup when we are sick may be much greater than that of similar soup from a can or mix. It could be the thought that counts; it could be a placebo response; but who is to say it is not some vibrational quality of food that scientific instruments of the present do not measure?

Orthodox Hindus place great importance on this quality. They consider the state of consciousness of the cook to be a great influence on the energetic nature of food and believe that, independent of its nutritional value, food can affect the state of consciousness of those who consume it, helping or hindering their spiritual development, by its energetic nature. They try to eat only freshly prepared food, disdaining reheated food, even if it tastes the same, because its energy is changed for the worse.

I would feel silly giving you rules about protecting the vibrational quality of food you buy and cook, but I would like you, at least, to think about this subject. We do not live by nutrients alone. As I wrote earlier, eating is a major source of pleasure, a primary focus of social interaction, a definer of individual and cultural identity, and an important influence on health. Think about the good feelings—of comfort, security, and love—that come from a meal prepared with care and love and eaten in the company of family and friends.*

It may be useful to keep some of this in mind when you shop for food, prepare it for the table, and select restaurants in which to eat. Pay attention to the feel of stores and restaurants and the people who manage them, to the aesthetic appearance of food, its freshness, colors, and odors, to your own attitudes about cleaning, cutting, and cooking the food you bring home. Enough said. I will conclude by quoting a verse from Lao Tzu:

> *If the sign of life is in your face*
> *He who responds to it*
> *Will feel secure and fit*
> *As, when in a friendly place,*
> *Sure of hearty care,*
> *A traveler gladly waits.*
> *Though it may not taste like food*
> *And he may not see the fare*
> *Or hear a sound of plates,*
> *How endless it is and how good!*

*Four films that beautifully portray this aspect of food are *Babette's Feast*, *Like Water for Chocolate*, *Big Night*, and *Eat Drink Man Woman*.

A HEALING STORY:
NOTHING IS EASY

AT SEVENTY-THREE, Jack Gumbin, a retired businessman in Tucson, Arizona, has a reputation for taking very good care of himself. A number of people who know him well told me how impressed they are with the attention he pays to his diet. In April 1983, Jack underwent coronary artery bypass surgery to take care of five obstructions in the blood vessels supplying his heart. Remarkably, his cardiac function has been fine since then, and the bypasses continue to function well.

"I never had a heart attack," Jack told me. Then he continued:

I'd been feeling fine. Then one day I played racquetball with a twenty-one-year-old. I suddenly felt tired and wanted to rest, but he didn't want to stop. I finished the game but then felt tired the whole weekend. The next week I went in for a cardiac stress test, the problem was discovered, and I had the surgery.

I never smoked and was never overweight. But I liked fatty foods and red meat. My favorite food was roast beef. I played racquetball once or twice a week, but otherwise wasn't getting any exercise. And I certainly had a lot of stress in my life.

When I recovered from the bypass surgery, I went to the University of Arizona to learn about changing my lifestyle, especially how to reduce stress and improve my diet to keep my arteries healthy. I did some psychological work, which helped. And I concentrated on cutting down significantly on red meat and fats. At that time my total cholesterol was 248 with HDL in the upper 30s. By changing how I ate, I got the total down to 200 and increased HDL to about 50. I was also taking niacin daily.

My wife strongly supported me with all these lifestyle changes, which was a big help. I like to eat out but rarely order red meat. I often eat fish and vegetables. I used to drink a lot of diluted coffee, but it was giving me headaches. Now I still drink weak coffee three or four days a week, but mostly I drink green tea, which I like. About a year ago I went on a cholesterol-lowering drug (lovastatin), and that has brought my cholesterol down even more. I also take Rythmol for an irregular heartbeat and a psyllium product every day along with vitamins C, E, and niacin and half an aspirin daily. And I do regular aerobic exercise, on a treadmill or elliptical trainer five days a week.

I asked Jack if these lifestyle changes had been easy.

"Nothing is easy," he replied. "But it's easy when your life is at stake."

7

AN ALCHEMIST
IN THE KITCHEN

I DISCOVERED the joy of cooking when I was in the clinical years of medical school. I found that working long hours among people who were stressed, anxious, and often unhappy in unpleasant surroundings put me, not surprisingly, in a bad state of mind. Also, there was nothing but dismal food to eat. At one of the prestigious Boston hospitals in which I worked, if medical students, interns, and residents missed cafeteria meals—a common occurrence on busy services—their only recourse was to go to a small, windowless room with vending machines for candy and soda and a table with the following items: a large plastic tub of peanut butter (the usual kind, full of partially hydrogenated oil), a plastic tub of jelly, and packages of saltine crackers.

Coming home from forty-eight- or seventy-two-hour stretches in this environment, I felt the need to detoxify on all levels. I would take a shower or bath, and then I would cook something good to eat. I found that preparing food took care of my mind and spirit. In the first place, it focused my awareness. Slicing and chopping have always been meditative for me, and so I prefer to do them by hand rather than using automated kitchen appliances. I like mastering various cutting techniques with good sharp knives, and the challenge of taking on a head of cabbage, a celery root, or a whole pineapple. I engage in this activity mindfully, bringing more of my consciousness to the present moment than usual. Awareness of the danger present in wielding sharp instruments helps concentrate my attention.

One of the great appeals of food preparation is that it is a way of creating order—for example, by reducing an ungainly vegetable to a neat mound of relatively equal pieces and by separating out any extraneous or unusable material. When I remove the outer leaves of a cabbage, peel onions, or cut away brown spots from fruits and vegetables, I am aware that I am sorting the good from the bad, saving all the best parts for incorporation into the meal and discarding the rest. I have seen many people throw away the big, tough stalks of broccoli, not realizing that they have delicious hearts. It takes just a few minutes and a bit of skill with a sharp knife to peel them, slicing beneath the fibrous outer layer to expose the tender interior. Cut into chunks and steamed or boiled along with the florets, broccoli stalks are wonderful. Of course, using them is also economical, since you get more out of the vegetable than if you just use the tops.

Besides making order, which can be a soothing remedy for a jangled mind, food preparation and cooking constitute a kind of practical magic that has great application to other areas of life. When you approach the raw ingredients of a dish, you have an idea in mind of what you want to create. That idea might be a visual picture or a verbal description. It might include imagined aromas and flavors. The task of the cook is to translate vision into reality, to manifest in the real world a creation that begins in the mind. What is that if not practical magic?

Cooking starts with imagination, with conceiving, picturing, and anticipating the look and smell and taste of something wonderful to eat. It then involves manipulation of a vast number of variables to bring the concept into reality. You cannot learn cooking from books, nor can recipes tell you how to do it well, no matter how detailed they are. You learn cooking by doing it, especially in the company of others more skilled than you, when you can pay attention to how dishes you like are prepared; then you can try them yourself and learn from your mistakes.

Good cooks are never dependent on cookbooks or recipes. They improvise, experiment, and feel free to change written instructions. Once you master the magical art of cooking, you can look at a recipe for inspiration, then let your own creativity take wing. You can add ingredients by handfuls, smatterings, and smidgeons rather than in measured amounts and can figure out how to compensate for a missing ingredient. You will know how to correct unbalanced flavors with spices and herbs by tasting rather than by referring to recipes.

You will have the ability to prepare a number of dishes that require different cooking methods and times and bring them all to perfection at the same moment.

I like to go into a strange kitchen and, working with whatever is in the refrigerator and pantry, create a meal that is delicious and healthful. I like shopping for food without any idea of what I am going to make and letting my plans for dinner be shaped by what looks best. If the organic broccoli is so appealingly green and fresh that I just have to buy it, I may make a main dish of it with pasta. If the salmon fillets look at their best, I buy them to poach or broil. If organic strawberries are available, they will be dessert that night.

Buying and preparing your own food also gives you the chance to influence the health of your whole family for the better. Creating family traditions of healthy eating is one of the most important things you can do for your children, whose food preferences will form early in life and who will be subjected to tremendous pressure from peers and from advertising to make unhealthy choices. Involve children in food preparation whenever they show interest; talk with them about food; and help them understand that healthy eating is the cornerstone of a healthy lifestyle, that it will make them strong and energetic and attractive. Teach them that even small changes in their diets can make big differences.

Once you understand the principles of cooking and have mastered the art of it, you can apply it in other situations. When I first went to South America to study medicinal plants in the 1960s, I spent time in the arid highlands of Peru, in an impoverished area where the range of available foods was limited. Often I was forced to eat in primitive roadside restaurants that served mainly rice, fried potatoes, and greasy stews full of chilies, tough chunks of meat, and overcooked vegetables. Occasionally, however, I would see a welcome sign—"*chifa*"—the Peruvian name for a Chinese restaurant. There are many fine Chinese restaurants in Lima and other coastal cities of Peru, but these simple, little places in the mountains were unusual, often run by descendants of Chinese workers imported to build the railroads in the high Andes.

What impressed me about these restaurants and why I was so happy to find them was that they served good food, made from the same local ingredients. It was not Chinese food as I knew it in North America—it had chilies, corn, and potatoes, for instance—but it was good. The meat, instead of being served in unappetizing hunks, was trimmed, finely cut, stir-fried with vegetables, and flavored well. I could order purely vegetarian dishes, too. These displaced chefs used principles of cooking from a highly developed cuisine, applied them to locally available ingredients, and created better menus than the indigenous restaurants of the region. This is one example of what I mean by taking the magical art of cooking with you.

Moreover, mastery of that art requires that you develop your powers of observation and the clarity of your imagination. You have to learn how to manage time, deal with unexpected developments, and not fall into states of frustration and despair when the objects of your efforts fail to develop the way you want them to. Being able to cook with other people is an ultimate test of human compatibility. In short, training in the kitchen is good preparation for life in general.

I do not mean to downplay the fact that cooking requires effort when I describe its rewards and pleasures. Clearly, for many people it is a chore and a bother, making fast food and processed food appear to be very attractive alternatives. I have had my share of unpleasant experiences making meals I was not motivated to make, and I know nothing more annoying than following recipes that don't work. The very worst recipes are complicated and laborious and then fail to produce promised results. I have tried my hand at preparing exotic dishes that required strange ingredients I never used before or since. Long ago I had a brief French cooking phase, and I once took a class in Chinese cooking. Today, my cooking is simple and efficient. Even when I am alone, I almost always cook from scratch. I like dishes that are quick and easy to make, call for ingredients I have on hand or are easy to get, and do not use up every pot and utensil in the kitchen. Of course, they must be healthful and delicious.

The recipes that follow produce those results. They fall within the guidelines of the optimum diet, as I have explained them in this book,* and I promise that they will produce satisfying results. Some are of my own invention, some are adaptations of recipes I have found elsewhere, and some were contributed by associates and friends. I have tested them all, eaten them all, and include them all in my own diet, some of them regularly. I hope you will like them as

*See Appendix A, page 261.

much as I do and will get from them a sense that preparing the right kind of food can be quick and easy, even fun. Feel free to experiment with these recipes and alter them to suit your own tastes.

You might have more fun doing this with others than by yourself. I invite you to visit my Web site (*www.drweil.com*) and chat with people who share an interest in eating well for optimum health. You can exchange ideas with them, develop further meal plans, and refine or improve upon these recipes. And enjoy!

A HEALING STORY: WHY I EAT HEALTHY

I THOUGHT IT would it would be interesting to interview my eight-year-old daughter Diana about her eating habits. Her half brothers and sister eat meat, but she does not, and she also stopped eating fish some time ago. I asked her to tell me why she follows this sort of diet and this is what she had to say:

I eat healthy because then I don't get sick. And I bet you live longer if you eat healthy and exercise.

I don't like to eat spicy stuff, and I don't like spinach or onions. I do like salad, broccoli, potatoes, rice, and pasta. I eat scrambled eggs, not a lot of them, and only the healthy kind of eggs—I forget what you call them. I also eat some cheese, but only certain kinds. I'm not crazy about tofu, but it's okay in soup. I like soyburgers, and I use soy milk on my cereal. I don't think I ever drank regular milk in my life. I love fruit and juice. And tomatoes and carrots. And homemade tomato sauce—that's what I like best on pasta.

I got interested in eating healthy because of you. And I did eat meat when I was really little, but one time someone gave me a hot dog and said, "Here's your pig sandwich." I never realized meat came from animals until then. When I did, I stopped eating it. I think I'm the only vegetarian in my class. About half of my friends are interested in eating healthy. I don't really know how to teach others about it, but if I knew I would. At least I would if I wouldn't hurt anybody's feelings or make anybody mad.

The only thing that makes me mad is when people say they're vegetarians, and they eat chicken or even hot dogs.

I never eat at fast-food places. The only time is maybe on a long road trip, when that's the only place to eat. I hardly ever have French fries, and if there's nothing else, I'll order a hamburger without the meat. When I go to restaurants, if they don't have healthy food, I'll get the healthiest thing I can find.

I'm very happy eating healthy. And, by the way, I like chocolate, some cookies, and a few kinds of lollipops.

8

THE RECIPES

AFTER EACH recipe you will find a nutritional analysis—per serving—that will help you estimate your daily caloric intake and its breakdown into macronutrients. (The values are always exclusive of any optional ingredients.) You will also find information about key nutritional benefits of these dishes. Note that I do not give sodium content for most of the recipes, since they direct you to add "salt to taste." Most of the sodium in the dishes will come from added salt or soy sauce; one teaspoon of salt provides 2,120 milligrams of sodium, and one tablespoon of reduced-sodium soy sauce provides 700 milligrams.

SOUPS

∞ Mushroom Barley Soup ∞

1 cup medium pearl barley
6 cups Vegetable Stock (see page 210)
1¼ cups onion, chopped
2 cloves garlic, minced
3 tablespoons extra-virgin olive oil
1 pound fresh mushrooms, sliced (shiitake, if possible)
4 tablespoons dry sherry
4 tablespoons reduced-sodium soy sauce, or to taste
2 teaspoons dried dill weed

1. Rinse and drain the barley. In a large pot, cook the barley, covered, in 1½ cups of the stock until tender.

2. Sauté the onions and garlic in the olive oil until they are translucent. Add the mushrooms and sherry and cook, uncovered, until the mushrooms are soft.

3. Add the mushroom mixture to the barley with the remaining stock and the rest of the ingredients. Bring the soup to a boil, reduce heat, cover, simmer for 20 minutes, and serve.

Servings: 4. Calories 590, fat 17 g (26% calories from fat), saturated fat 3 g, protein 18 g, carbohydrate 91 g, cholesterol 4 mg, sodium 700 mg, fiber 12 g

Nutritional benefits: Unrefined, whole grain; monounsaturated fat; micronutrients, including immune-enhancing polysaccharides in shiitake mushrooms

∞ *Vegetable Stock* ∞

1 tablespoon extra-virgin olive oil
2 leeks, white and light-green parts only, well washed and chopped
4 medium onions, chopped
6 large carrots, peeled and chopped
3 stalks celery, chopped
1 small bunch parsley stems
2 teaspoons whole dried marjoram
½ teaspoon whole dried thyme
3 bay leaves (Turkish) or ½ bay leaf (California)
1½ gallons cold water

1. Heat the olive oil over medium-high heat in a large pot, add the vegetables, and stir-fry to brown lightly.

2. Add the herbs and cold water. Bring to a boil, reduce heat, and simmer, partly covered, for 1 hour.

3. Strain the stock through a fine sieve or cheesecloth-lined colander. Cool and chill or freeze for later use.

Servings: 20. Calories 36, fat less than 1 g, saturated fat 0 g, protein less than 1 g, carbohydrate 7 g, cholesterol 0 g, sodium 25 mg, fiber 2 g

Nutritional benefits: Micronutrients

∞ Asparagus Soup ∞

3½ pounds fresh asparagus
3 large yellow onions, chopped
2 tablespoons extra-virgin olive oil
10 cups Vegetable Stock (see page 210)
salt and black pepper to taste

1. Cut off and discard the tough ends of the asparagus. Cut off the top 3 inches of the stalks and set aside. Cut the bottoms of the stalks into 1-inch pieces.

2. Sauté the onions in olive oil until they are soft and golden.

3. In a large pot, heat the stock, and add the cooked onions and the 1-inch pieces of asparagus stalks. Simmer, covered, until the asparagus is soft.

4. Purée the soup in a food processor. Return it to the pot, season to taste with salt and pepper, and add the asparagus tops. Cook until the asparagus tops are just tender, about 5 minutes. Soup can be served hot or chilled.

Servings: 8. Calories 275, fat 8.5 g (27% of calories from fat), saturated fat 2 g, protein 10 g, carbohydrate 41.5 g, cholesterol 3 mg, fiber 4.5 g
Nutritional benefits: Micronutrients; monounsaturated fat

∞ Quick Creamy Tomato Soup ∞

1 large onion, chopped
1 tablespoon extra-virgin olive oil
3 pounds fresh, ripe Italian tomatoes, chopped (about 6 cups)
8 sun-dried tomatoes, soaked
1 cup soy milk
salt and black and red pepper to taste
3 tablespoons fresh parsley, basil, or dill, chopped

1. In a large pot, sauté the onions in the olive oil until they are soft, then add the fresh tomatoes and stir until the mixture boils.

2. Remove the dried tomatoes from their soaking water and chop them coarsely. Add them and their soaking water to the pot and cook, stirring to prevent sticking.

3. Reduce heat to low, cover, and simmer for 30 minutes. Add the soy milk and season to taste with salt and black and red pepper.

4. Serve in bowls with the chopped green herbs as garnish.

Servings: 3. Calories 196, fat 7.5 g (31% of calories from fat), saturated fat 1 g, protein 7.1 g, carbohydrate 30 g, cholesterol 0 mg, fiber 8 g

Nutritional benefits: Monounsaturated fat; micronutrients, including lycopene from tomatoes and isoflavones from soy

∽ *Roasted Vegetable Soup* ∽

3 large carrots, peeled and coarsely chopped
3 stalks celery, trimmed and roughly cut
1 large onion, roughly cut
1 tablespoon extra-virgin olive oil
8 cloves garlic, coarsely chopped
4 cups water
¼ cup dried mushroom pieces (Italian porcini, if possible)
¼ teaspoon dried thyme
salt and black or red pepper to taste

1. Preheat oven to 500°F. Place the carrots, celery, and onion in a small (8 x 8 inch) nonstick pan or dish with the olive oil. Toss to coat the vegetables. Bake for 10 minutes.

2. Remove pan from oven, add the garlic, and toss again. Bake for another 10–15 minutes until the vegetables are browned.

3. Remove pan from oven, add 1 cup of water and stir to loosen any vegetables that may be stuck. Pour this into a pot with the remaining ingredients. Bring to a boil, reduce heat, cover, and simmer for 30 minutes.

4. Season to taste with salt and black or red pepper, and serve or use as the base for other soups, stews, or pasta dishes.

Servings: 4. Calories 239, fat 5 g (19% of calories from fat), saturated fat 1 g, protein 8 g, carbohydrate 42 g, cholesterol 3 mg, fiber 5 g

Nutritional benefits: Monounsaturated fat; micronutrents, including carotenoids in carrots

∞ Yellow Pepper and Carrot Soup ∞

2½ tablespoons extra-virgin olive oil
3 large carrots, peeled and cut in rounds
1 cup leeks, white part only, washed and cut in ½-inch pieces
1 large yellow pepper, seeded, and cut in 1-inch squares
3 sprigs fresh rosemary
a pinch of ground cumin
3½ cups Vegetable Stock (see page 210)
salt and black pepper to taste

1. In a large pot, heat the olive oil over medium heat, add the carrots, leeks, pepper, rosemary, and cumin, stir well, cover, and cook for 10 minutes.

2. Add the stock, and season to taste with salt and pepper. Simmer uncovered for 20 minutes or until the carrots are tender.

3. Remove the rosemary, and purée the soup in a food processor.
Servings: 4. Calories 290, fat 13 g (38% of calories from fat), saturated fat 2 g, protein 7 g, carbohydrate 40 g, cholesterol 2 mg, fiber 5 g
Nutritional benefits: Micronutrients, including carotenoids; mono-unsaturated fat

∞ Zucchini Watercress Soup ∞

4 tablespoons extra-virgin olive oil
2 cups yellow onions, finely chopped
3 cups Vegetable Stock (see page 210)
2 pounds zucchini (about 4 medium), scrubbed well, and coarsely chopped
4 cups (loosely packed) watercress, washed well, large stems removed
salt and freshly ground black pepper to taste
fresh lemon juice to taste

1. Heat the olive oil in a large pot, add the onions, cover, and cook over low heat, stirring occasionally, until the onions are tender and lightly colored, about 25 minutes.

2. Add the stock and bring to a boil.

3. Add the zucchini and return to a boil. Lower heat, cover, and simmer about 20 minutes.

4. Remove the soup from heat, add the watercress, cover, and let stand for 5 minutes.

5. Pour the soup through a colander, reserving the liquid. Put the solids in a food processor with 1 cup of the reserved liquid and purée.

6. Return the purée to the cooking pot and add additional liquid (about 2 cups) until the soup is the consistency you want.

7. Season to taste with the salt, pepper, and lemon juice, and simmer briefly to heat through.

Servings: 4. Calories 309, fat 17 g (47% of calories from fat), saturated fat 3 g, protein 9 g, carbohydrate 34 g, cholesterol 2 mg, fiber 6 g
Nutritional benefits: Micronutrients; monounsaturated fat

∽ *Smoky Red Bean Soup* ∽

1 pound dried red beans
6 fresh plum tomatoes, peeled, seeded, and diced (see Step 2)
1 tablespoon extra-virgin olive oil
1 large onion, chopped
6 cloves garlic, minced
8 cups water
1 package (6 ounces) baked, pressed tofu (smoke flavor), diced
salt and red pepper to taste

1. Rinse the beans and allow them to soak in cold water for 8 hours. Drain.

2. Dip the tomatoes in boiling water for 15 seconds, cool, and peel. Cut the tomatoes in half, squeeze out the seeds and discard. Dice the tomatoes.

3. In a large soup pot, heat the olive oil over medium heat, add the onions and garlic, and sauté until soft.

4. Raise heat to high, add the beans and water, cover, and bring to a boil. Reduce heat, add the tomatoes, and simmer the beans 2–3 hours until desired tenderness.

5. Add the tofu, season to taste with salt and red pepper, and heat through.

Servings: 8. Calories 250, fat 3 g (10% of calories from fat), saturated fat 1.4 g, protein 17 g, carbohydrate 40 g, cholesterol 0 mg, fiber 16 g

Nutritional benefits: Monounsaturated fat; micronutrients, including high fiber and low-glycemic-index carbohydrate in beans and isoflavones in tofu

∞ *Winter Root Soup* ∞

2 boiling potatoes
2 medium parsnips
2 large carrots
1 turnip
1 rutabaga
2 tablespoons extra-virgin olive oil
1 large onion, sliced
2 cloves garlic
1 bay leaf (Turkish, not California)
½ teaspoon each dried whole thyme and marjoram
1 teaspoon dried basil
6 cups water or Vegetable Stock (see page 210)
1 cup dry white vermouth
salt and black pepper to taste
1 bunch fresh parsley, stems removed, chopped
1 cup freshly grated Parmesan cheese

1. Peel all the vegetables and cut them into bite-size pieces.

2. Heat the olive oil in a soup pot, add the onion, and cook until translucent.

3. Add the vegetables and sauté until they begin to color.

4. Add the garlic and dried herbs.

5. Add the water or stock, the vermouth, and salt and pepper to taste. Bring to a boil, cover, reduce heat, and simmer until vegetables are tender, about 30 minutes. Remove the bay leaf and correct seasoning.

6. Serve in bowls sprinkled with the chopped parsley and pass the grated Parmesan cheese as an accompaniment.

Servings: 6. Calories 468, fat 13 g (26% of calories from fat), saturated fat 4 g, protein 15.5 g, carbohydrate 65 g, cholesterol 13 mg, fiber 7 g

Nutritional benefits: Micronutrients

∞ *Winter Squash Soup* ∞

1 tablespoon dark (roasted) sesame oil
2 large onions, chopped
1 pound winter squash (buttercup, kabocha, butternut), peeled, seeded,
and diced (about 2 heaping cups)
4 tablespoons whole-wheat pastry flour
6 cups Vegetable Stock (see page 210)
salt to taste
1 cup soy milk (optional)

1. In a soup pot, heat the sesame oil over medium heat and sauté the onions until translucent. Add the squash and cook it with the onions, stirring, for 5 minutes.

2. Add the flour, and sauté for 2 minutes more. Don't worry if some of the flour sticks to the pot.

3. Add the vegetable stock, stir well, cover, and bring mixture to a boil, then reduce heat and simmer until the squash is soft, about 45 minutes. Add salt to taste.

4. Purée the mixture in a food processor, then return it to pot. Correct seasoning. Add the soy milk, if desired, and serve.

Servings: 6. Calories 262, fat 7 g (24% of calories from fat), saturated fat 1.5 g, protein 9.5 g, carbohydrate 42 g, cholesterol 3 mg, fiber 4 g

Nutritional benefits: Micronutrients, including carotenoids in squash and isoflavones in soy milk

∞ *Summer Melon Soup* ∞

1 ripe cantaloupe, rind and seeds removed, diced, about 4 cups
an equal amount of watermelon, seeded and diced
juice of 1 fresh lemon
1–2 teaspoons honey, liquefied (20 seconds in microwave)
¼ teaspoon salt
2 fresh jalapeño peppers, seeded and finely minced
½ cup fresh blueberries

1. Purée the cantaloupe and watermelon together. Flavor to taste with the lemon juice, honey, and salt. Add the minced peppers. Chill.

2. Garnish servings of soup with a few blueberries.

Servings: 6. Calories 95, fat less than 1 g (7% of calories from fat), saturated fat less than 1 g, protein 2 g, carbohydrate 24 g, cholesterol 0 mg, sodium 103 mg, fiber 2 g

Nutritional benefits: Micronutrients

∽ Pasta Fagiole ∾
(White Bean & Pasta Soup)

1 cup dried small white beans
1 tablespoon extra-virgin olive oil
1 large onion, chopped
6 cloves garlic, minced
10 cups water or Vegetable Stock (see page 210)
½ teaspoon dried rosemary, crushed
1 cup small pasta, such as orzo or small shells
salt and black pepper to taste
2 tablespoons fresh parsley, chopped (optional)
1 cup freshly grated Parmesan cheese
additional extra-virgin olive oil (optional)

1. Wash the beans and allow them to soak in cold water for 8 hours. Drain.

2. In a large soup pot, heat 1 tablespoon of olive oil over medium heat, add the onion and garlic, and sauté until soft.

3. Raise heat to high, add the beans and water or stock, cover, and bring to a boil. Reduce heat to low, add the rosemary, and simmer 2 hours or until the beans are of desired tenderness.

4. Raise heat to high, add the pasta, and boil it until it is *al dente*.

5. Season the soup to taste with salt and pepper, garnish with the chopped parsley, if desired, and serve accompanied by grated Parmesan cheese and the optional extra-virgin olive oil.

Servings: 6. Calories 346, fat 11 g (29% of calories from fat), saturated fat 2.5 g, protein 15 g, carbohydrate 47 g, cholesterol 5 mg, fiber 10 g

Nutritional benefits: Monounsaturated fat; micronutrients, including fiber in beans

SALADS

❧ *Middle Eastern Chopped Salad* ❧

1 cucumber, peeled, seeded, and diced
2 fresh tomatoes, seeded and diced
2 scallions, trimmed and chopped
1 sweet yellow pepper, seeded and chopped
3 tablespoons black olives (Kalamata or oil-cured, if possible),
pitted and chopped
2 tablespoons fresh parsley, chopped
3 tablespoons fresh lemon juice
2 tablespoons extra-virgin olive oil
salt and black pepper to taste
1/4 cup feta cheese, crumbled (optional)

1. Combine all the ingredients.
2. Season to taste with salt and pepper, and serve.

Servings: 4. Calories 116, fat 6 g (40% of calories from fat), saturated fat 1.5 g, protein 4 g, carbohydrate 15 g, cholesterol 8 mg, fiber 4 g
Nutritional benefits: Monounsaturated fat; micronutrients

❧ *Turkish Spinach Salad* ❧

1 pound fresh spinach, washed, stems removed
2 fresh tomatoes, sliced
6 scallions, trimmed and thinly sliced
5 tablespoons plain yogurt, nonfat or low-fat
2 tablespoons extra-virgin olive oil
2 garlic cloves, minced
1/2 teaspoon dried thyme
salt and black pepper to taste

1. Dry the spinach, tear it into large pieces, and combine it with the tomatoes and scallions in a bowl.
2. Combine the yogurt, olive oil, minced garlic, and thyme, adding salt and pepper to taste.

3. Add the yogurt mixture to the vegetables and mix well. Season to taste with salt and pepper.

Servings: 4. Calories 124, fat 8 g (52% of calories from fat), saturated fat 1 g, protein 5 g, carbohydrate 11.5 g, cholesterol 2 mg, fiber 5 g

Nutritional benefits: Monounsaturated fat; micronutrients; protein and calcium in yogurt

∞ *Lentil Salad* ∞

1 cup lentils (regular or French green)
6 sprigs fresh parsley
bay leaf (Turkish)
a pinch of dried thyme
2 tablespoons wine vinegar
2 scallions, minced
1 teaspoon dry mustard powder
salt and black pepper to taste
1/3 cup walnut oil
3 tablespoons fresh parsley, chopped

1. Soak the lentils in enough cold water to cover for 2 hours. Drain and place in a saucepan with the parsley sprigs, the bay leaf, and the thyme. Add boiling water to cover, and simmer for 35–45 minutes, covered, until tender. Drain and discard the parsley sprigs and bay leaf.

2. In a salad bowl, whisk together the wine vinegar, scallions, mustard, salt, and pepper. Add the walnut oil in a stream while whisking.

3. Add the lentils and toss with the dressing. Add the chopped fresh parsley. Correct the seasoning. Serve warm or cold.

Servings: 4. Calories 346, fat 19 g (48% of calories from fat), saturated fat 2 g, protein 15 g, carbohydrate 32 g, cholesterol 0 mg, fiber 16.5 g

Nutritional benefits: Protein, good carbohydrate, fiber from lentils; omega-3 fatty acids from walnut oil

✒ *Robust Beet Salad* ✒

3 pounds beets
¼ cup brown sugar
¼ cup rice or cider vinegar
¼ cup water
1 teaspoon wasabi powder (Japanese horseradish)
1 teaspoon dry mustard powder
1 large onion, sliced thin
salt to taste

1. Cut off the beet tops about an inch above the root. In a large pot cover the beets with three inches of cold water and bring to a boil. Cover pot and boil the beets over medium heat until tender, about 45 minutes.

2. Drain the beets and under cool running water slip off their skins. Trim off stems and root ends and slice the beets thinly.

3. Combine the sliced beets in a bowl with all the other ingredients, add salt to taste, and chill. Stir several times. This salad will keep for a week in the refrigerator.

Servings: 4. Calories 184, fat less than 1 g (2% of calories from fat), saturated fat less than 1 g, protein 4 g, carbohydrate 39 g, cholesterol 0 mg, fiber 7 g

Nutritional benefits: Micronutrients

✒ *Tunisian Salad* ✒

2 ripe tomatoes, peeled, seeded, and finely diced (about ¾ cup)
½ cucumber, peeled, seeded, and finely diced (about 1 cup)
1 small green apple, peeled, cored, and finely diced (about 1 cup)
2 tablespoons fresh, hot green chilies, seeded and finely chopped
4 scallions, trimmed and finely sliced
juice of ½ lemon
2 tablespoons extra-virgin olive oil
1 tablespoon dried spearmint leaves, pressed through a fine sieve
salt and black pepper to taste

1. Combine all the ingredients in a shallow serving bowl. Mix well and season to taste.

2. Chill for 1 hour before serving.

Servings: 4. Calories 114, fat 7 g (49% of calories from fat), saturated fat 1 g, protein 2 g, carbohydrate 14.5 g, cholesterol 0 mg, fiber 3 g

Nutritional benefits: Monounsaturated fat; micronutrients

✐ Orange-Jicama Salad ✐

4 cups jicama, peeled and julienned
2 oranges, sectioned
2 tablespoons fresh coriander (cilantro), chopped
$1/3$ cup fresh orange juice
2 tablespoons balsamic vinegar
1 tablespoon extra-virgin olive oil
salt and black pepper to taste

1. Mix the jicama, orange sections, and chopped coriander in a bowl.

2. Whisk together the remaining ingredients, toss with the jicama-orange mixture, season to taste with salt and pepper, and serve.

Servings: 4. Calories 107, fat 4 g (29% of calories from fat), saturated fat 0.5 g, protein 2 g, carbohydrate 18 g, cholesterol 0 mg, fiber 7 g

Nutritional benefits: Monounsaturated fat; micronutrients

✐ Cucumber Raita ✐

2 large cucumbers, peeled, seeded, and chopped
1 medium onion, finely chopped
1 tablespoon salt
2 cups plain, nonfat yogurt
$1/2$ teaspoon ground cumin
black pepper to taste

1. Mix the cucumbers, onion, and salt in a bowl. Let stand for $1/2$ hour.

2. Drain off liquid, rinse well with cold water, and drain; then soak in cold water to remove as much salt as desired. Drain well.

3. Add the yogurt, cumin, and pepper. Refrigerate for at least 2 hours before serving.

Servings: 4. Calories 109, fat 0.5 g (4% of calories from fat), saturated fat 0 g, protein 8.5 g, carbohydrate 19.5 g, cholesterol 3 mg, fiber 3 g

Nutritional benefits: Protein and calcium from yogurt

෨ Cranberry Wheatberry Salad ෨

1 cup wheatberries (whole-wheat grains)
½ cup dried cranberries
1 tablespoon extra-virgin olive oil
juice of 1 orange with pulp
juice of ½ lemon
salt to taste
¼ cup oil-cured olives, pitted and chopped (optional)

1. Place the wheatberries in a pot with 4 cups of cold water. Bring to a boil, cover, reduce heat, and boil gently for about 1 hour until the wheatberries are chewy-tender. Drain.

2. Toss the warm wheatberries together with the remaining ingredients. Allow to cool, then add salt to taste.

Servings: 4. Calories 209, fat 4.5 g (18% of calories from fat), saturated fat 0.5 g, protein 6.5 g, carbohydrate 39.5 g, cholesterol 0 mg, fiber 8 g

Nutritional benefits: Unrefined grain; micronutrients

෨ Basic Tossed Salad ෨

8 cups mixed salad greens, washed and dried
2 tablespoons extra-virgin olive oil
salt and black pepper to taste
2 teaspoons balsamic vinegar
1 clove garlic (optional)

1. Place the salad greens in a large bowl. Add enough olive oil to coat the greens lightly but thoroughly. Toss well.

2. Add salt and pepper to taste and a little vinegar. Toss again and taste to determine if you need more vinegar or seasoning. Toss well.

3. If you use the garlic, crush it into the first portion of vinegar added.

4. Serve salad immediately.

Servings: 4. Calories 40, fat 3.5 g (73.5% of calories from fat), saturated fat 0.5 g, protein 1 g, carbohydrate 2 g, cholesterol 0 mg, fiber 1 g

Nutritional benefits: Monounsaturated fat; micronutrients, including fiber and protective phytochemicals

◎ *Citrus Dressing for Salad* ◎

⅓ cup fresh orange or grapefruit juice
2 tablespoons balsamic vinegar
1 tablespoon extra-virgin olive oil
salt and black pepper to taste

1. Whisk all the ingredients together and use on salads of your choice.

Servings: 3. Calories 54, fat 5 g (74% of calories from fat), saturated fat 1 g, protein less than 1 g, carbohydrate 3.5 g, cholesterol 0 mg, fiber 0 g

Nutritional benefits: Monounsaturated fat; micronutrients

◎ *Green Garlic Dressing* ◎

½ cup (4 ounces) silken tofu
2 tablespoons extra-virgin olive oil
1 tablespoon fresh lemon juice
1 clove garlic
¼ cup (packed) fresh coriander (cilantro) leaves or parsley leaves
salt and black and red pepper to taste

1. Place all the ingredients in a food processor or blender and process until smooth.

2. Use on salads, vegetables, or fish.

Servings: 4. Calories 86, fat 8 g (83% of calories from fat), saturated fat 1 g, protein 3 g, carbohydrate 1 g, cholesterol 0 mg, fiber less than 1 g

Nutritional benefits: Protein, calcium, isoflavones from tofu; mono-unsaturated fat; micronutrients

✆ *Dressing for Cole Slaw* ✆

½ cup (4 ounces) silken tofu
2 tablespoons extra-virgin olive oil
1 tablespoon cider vinegar
1 tablespoon Dijon mustard
1 teaspoon honey
½ teaspoon poppy seeds
salt and black pepper to taste

1. Combine all the ingredients in a food processor or blender and process until smooth. Season to taste with salt and pepper.

Servings: 4. Calories 94, fat 9 g (78% of calories from fat), saturated fat 1 g, protein 3 g, carbohydrate 3 g, cholesterol 0 mg, fiber less than 1 g

Nutritional benefits: Protein, calcium, and isoflavones from soy; monounsaturated fat

✆ *Tartar Sauce* ✆

½ cup (4 ounces) silken tofu
2 tablespoons extra-virgin olive oil
1 tablespoon fresh lemon juice
1 tablespoon onion, chopped
1 tablespoon dill pickle, finely chopped
1 tablespoon capers
salt and black or red pepper to taste

1. Place the tofu, olive oil, lemon juice, and onion in a food processor or blender, and process until smooth.

2. Scrape the mixture into a bowl, add the dill pickle and capers, and season to taste with salt and black or red pepper.

3. Serve on fish or vegetables.

Servings: 4. Calories 90, fat 8 g (79% of calories from fat), saturated fat 1 g, protein 3 g, carbohydrate 2.5 g, cholesterol 0 mg, fiber less than 1 g

Nutritional benefits: Protein, calcium, and isoflavones from soy; monounsaturated fat

✆ Pickled Carrots ✆

3 cloves garlic, minced
1 tablespoon onion, coarsely chopped
3 tablespoons extra-virgin olive oil
¼ cup wine vinegar
½ teaspoon dry mustard powder
1 tablespoon whole mixed pickling spices, tied in cheesecloth
salt and black pepper to taste
1 pound carrots, peeled and cut into matchsticks
1 small onion, thinly sliced

1. Sauté the garlic and chopped onion in the olive oil until almost tender, about 5 minutes.

2. Stir in the wine vinegar, dry mustard, pickling spices, salt, pepper, and carrots. Simmer, covered, for 5 minutes. The carrots should be very crunchy. Remove from heat.

3. Remove the cheesecloth with the spices. Transfer the carrot mixture to a shallow dish. Top with the thinly sliced onion. Cover and refrigerate until needed, stirring occasionally.

4. Serve cold as an appetizer.

Servings: 4. Calories 212, fat 11 g (43% of calories from fat), saturated fat 1.5 g, protein 3 g, carbohydrate 30 g, cholesterol 0 mg, fiber 5 g

Nutritional benefits: Micronutrients

ஒ   *Indian Onion Relish*   ஒ

1 large red onion, diced
1 tablespoon extra-virgin olive oil
1 tablespoon paprika
1 tablespoon brown sugar
1 teaspoon turmeric
2 tablespoons fresh lemon or lime juice
1/4 teaspoon red pepper
salt to taste

1. Soak the onions in cold water for about 10 minutes and drain. Repeat several times to get rid of their sharpness.

2. Combine the onions with the remaining ingredients. Add salt to taste.

3. Serve as a condiment to rice dishes, or on sandwiches.

Servings: 4. Calories 54, fat 4 g (57% of calories from fat), protein 1 g, carbohydrate 5.5 g, cholesterol 0 mg, fiber 1 g

Nutritional benefits: Monounsaturated fat; micronutrients; no saturated fat

APPETIZERS

ஒ   *Garlic Dip or Sauce*   ஒ

3 slices whole-wheat toast
1/4 cup walnuts
4 cloves garlic, mashed
2 tablespoons fresh lemon juice
1 tablespoon extra-virgin olive oil
3/4 cup water
2 tablespoons fresh parsley leaves
salt and pepper to taste

1. Place the toast in a food processor and process into fine crumbs.

2. With the motor running, add the walnuts and garlic and process until they are ground fine.

3. Add the remaining ingredients with the motor running and process until smooth, adding more water if the mixture seems too thick.

4. Scrape the mixture into a bowl, and season to taste with salt and pepper.

Servings: 4. Calories 166, fat 10 g (49% of calories from fat), saturated fat 1.5 g, protein 6 g, carbohydrate 18 g, cholesterol 0 mg, fiber 3 g

Nutritional benefits: Omega-3 fatty acids from walnuts; monounsaturated micronutrients, including fat; fiber from whole-wheat bread

∽ Eggplant-Walnut Paté ∾

1 large eggplant
1 cup walnut pieces
2 teaspoons fresh gingerroot, peeled, grated, and finely chopped
2 cloves garlic, mashed
1 tablespoon extra-virgin olive oil
1/8 teaspoon ground allspice
salt and hot pepper sauce to taste

1. Preheat oven to 450°F. Pierce the eggplant with a fork in several places and bake until very soft, about 45 minutes.

2. While the eggplant is baking, grind the walnuts in a food processor until very fine, and set aside.

3. Remove the eggplant from oven, slash to let steam escape, drain off any liquid, and scrape the pulp into a food processor with the gingerroot, garlic, and olive oil. Process until smooth.

4. Add the ground walnuts, and process until smooth.

5. Flavor the mixture with the allspice, salt, and drops of hot pepper sauce to taste. Chill.

Servings: 8. Calories 126, fat 11 g (70% of calories from fat), saturated fat 1 g, protein 4.5 g, carbohydrate 6 g, cholesterol 0 mg, fiber 2 g

Nutritional benefits: Omega-3 fatty acids from walnuts; monounsaturated fat; micronutrients

❧   Bean Dip with Horseradish · ❧

2 cups cooked beans (cannelini, pinto, or Great Northern)
2 tablespoons extra-virgin olive oil
1 tablespoon prepared horseradish
2 scallions, trimmed and minced
salt to taste

1. Combine beans, olive oil, horseradish, and scallions in a blender or food processor and blend until smooth, adding a little water if necessary.

2. Season with salt to taste.

Servings: 8. Calories 94, fat 3.5 g (33% of calories from fat), saturated fat less than 1 g, protein 4.5 g, carbohydrate 12 g, cholesterol 0 mg, fiber 4 g

Nutritional benefits: Good carbohydrate; monounsaturated fat; micronutrients

❧   Lentil Walnut Spread   ❧

1 cup lentils
½ cup walnuts, chopped
2 teaspoons Dijon mustard
1 tablespoon red wine vinegar
salt and black or red pepper to taste

1. Wash the lentils, cover with cold water, bring to a boil, and cook until soft, about 1 hour.

2. Drain the lentils and combine with the remaining ingredients in a food processor. Blend until smooth, adding water as necessary to achieve a spreadable consistency.

3. Correct seasoning.

Servings: 8. Calories 130, fat 4.7 g (31% of calories from fat), saturated fat less than 1 g, protein 8.7 g, carbohydrate 15 g, cholesterol 0 mg, fiber 7.5 g

Nutritional benefits: Good carbohydrate; omega-3 fatty acids from walnuts; micronutrients

⌘ Sardine or Kipper Sandwich Spread ⌘

1 can sardines packed in water, or kipper snacks
1–2 teaspoons Dijon mustard
1 tablespoon onion, finely chopped
½ teaspoon fresh lemon juice

1. Drain the fish and mash them with a fork in a bowl together with the mustard.

2. Add the onion and lemon juice.

Servings: 1. Calories 202, fat 13.5 g (56% of calories from fat), saturated fat 2 g, protein 19.5 g, carbohydrate 2 g, cholesterol 60.5 mg, sodium 516 mg, fiber less than 1 g

Nutritional benefits: Protein and omega-3 fatty acids from fish

⌘ Hummus ⌘

1¾ cups dried chickpeas (garbanzos)
1 teaspoon baking soda
½ cup sesame tahini
¼ cup cold water
¼ cup fresh lemon juice
½ teaspoon ground cumin
3–4 cloves garlic, mashed
1 tablespoon extra-virgin olive oil

1. Soak the chickpeas for 8 hours with the baking soda in cold water to cover.

2. Bring the chickpeas to a boil over high heat, reduce heat, cover, and cook until soft, about 45 minutes. Drain, reserving a bit of the liquid.

3. Make the tahini sauce: Blend in a food processor or blender the tahini, cold water, lemon juice, cumin, and garlic. Measure out ½ cup of this sauce for the hummus, saving the rest.

4. Put the drained chickpeas in a food processor and process to a rough purée, adding a little of the cooking liquid if necessary. The mixture should not be totally smooth. Add the tahini sauce and process until just mixed.

5. Scrape the mixture into a bowl. Stir in the olive oil.

6. Serve with pita bread, whole-grain crackers, or carrot sticks.

Servings: 4. Calories 536, fat 24 g (39% of calories from fat), saturated fat 3 g, protein 23 g, carbohydrate 63 g, cholesterol 0 mg, fiber 17 g

Nutritional benefits: Protein, fiber, and good carbohydrate from chickpeas; fiber, calcium, and essential fatty acids from sesame seeds; monounsaturated fat

FISH

∽ *Mediterranean Tuna Steaks* ∽

2 ahi tuna steaks, 4–6 ounces each, about 1 inch thick
2 teaspoons extra-virgin olive oil
salt and pepper to taste
1 medium ripe tomato, diced fine
6 green olives, pitted and chopped
1 tablespoon scallions, chopped
2 teaspoons capers
1 clove garlic, mashed
a pinch of dried whole oregano

1. Rinse the tuna steaks under cold running water and pat dry. Brush them with 1 teaspoon of the olive oil and season them with salt and pepper.

2. Preheat grill or broiler. Meanwhile, mix all the remaining ingredients, season with salt and pepper, and set aside.

2. Grill the steaks on high heat or broil, about 2–3 minutes per side or until desired doneness.

3. Cover the steaks with topping mixture, and serve. Good hot or cold.

Servings: 2. Calories 161, fat 7 g (40% of calories from fat), saturated fat 1 g, protein 20.5 g, carbohydrate 3 g, cholesterol 38 mg, fiber 1 g

Nutritional benefits: Protein from fish

∾ Dill-Poached Fish Fillets ∾

¾ pound very thin fresh fish fillets, such as cod or Dover sole
salt and black pepper to taste
½ cup fresh dill weed, chopped
1 tablespoon fresh lemon juice
3 tablespoons water

1. Rinse the fillets under cold running water and pat dry.
2. Season the fillets with salt and pepper and sprinkle the dill over them.
3. Roll up the fillets and place them in a glass pie plate or ceramic dish with the lemon juice and water.
4. Microwave on high for 2 minutes. Turn the fillets and microwave for 1 minute more.
5. Serve warm or cold with Tartar Sauce (see page 224) or Green Garlic Dressing (see page 223).

Servings: 2. Calories 71, fat 0.5 g (7% of calories from fat), saturated fat 0 g, protein 15 g, carbohydrate 1 g, cholesterol 37 mg, fiber 0 g
Nutritional benefits: Protein from fish

∾ Pan-Fried Fish Fillets with Mushrooms ∾

2 teaspoons extra-virgin olive oil
¾ pound fish fillets, such as cod, halibut, or sole
salt and black pepper to taste
½ pound fresh mushrooms, such as oyster, shiitake, or portobello, sliced
2 scallions, trimmed and thinly sliced
2 fresh lemon wedges

1. Heat the olive oil in a skillet and cook the fish, about 2½ minutes on each side. Season with salt and pepper and remove it to a warm plate.
2. Add the mushrooms to the pan and cook them until they begin to brown. Season them to taste with salt and pepper.
3. Sprinkle the scallions on the fish and serve it with the mushrooms and lemon wedges.

Servings: 2. Calories 207, fat 6 g (27% of calories from fat), saturated fat less than 1 g, protein 32.5 g, carbohydrate 5 g, cholesterol 73 mg, fiber 1.4 g

Nutritional benefits: Protein from fish; monounsaturated fat; micronutrients

❧ Horseradish-Crusted Fish Fillets ❧

8–12 ounces fish, such as cod or halibut
½ cup dry whole-grain breadcrumbs
2–3 tablespoons prepared horseradish
2 tablespoons extra-virgin olive oil
salt and black pepper to taste

1. Preheat oven to 350°F. Rinse the fish under cold running water and pat dry.
2. Combine the remaining ingredients and press the mixture on top of the fish.
3. Bake the fish for 15 minutes or until desired doneness.
4. Place the fish under the broiler briefly to brown the crust.

Servings: 2. Calories 377, fat 17 g (40% of calories from fat), saturated fat 2.5 g, protein 34 g, carbohydrate 22 g, cholesterol 73 mg, fiber 2 g

Nutritional benefits: Protein from fish; monounsaturated fat

❧ Potato-Rosemary–Crusted Fish Fillets ❧

8–12 ounces thick fish fillet, such as cod or halibut
1 medium potato
salt and black pepper to taste
¼ teaspoon dried rosemary leaves, crushed
1 tablespoon extra-virgin olive oil

1. Rinse the fish under cold running water and pat dry.
2. Peel the potato and grate on the large holes of a grater. Squeeze excess water out of potato by pressing between sheets of paper towel.

3. Season the potato with salt, pepper, and rosemary and press it around the fish.

4. Heat a nonstick frying pan over medium high heat and add olive oil. Gently slide in fish. Cook for 3 minutes. Turn, using two spatulas, and cook for 3 minutes more.

Servings: 2. Calories 341, fat 8 g (21.5% of calories from fat), saturated fat 1 g, protein 34 g, carbohydrate 32 g, cholesterol 73 mg, fiber 3 g

Nutritional benefits: Protein from fish; monounsaturated fat

∽ Easy Poached Salmon ∽

fresh salmon fillets (allow 6 ounces per person)
1 carrot, peeled and sliced
1 small onion, sliced
1 stalk celery, sliced
2 slices lemon
several sprigs parsley
6 bay leaves (Turkish) or ½ bay leaf (California)
12 black peppercorns
salt to taste
1 cup dry white wine
juice of ½ lemon

1. Rinse the salmon fillets under cold water and cut them into individual portions.

2. Place in a large pot the carrot, onion, celery, lemon slices, parsley, bay leaves, and peppercorns.

3. Add the fish, cold water to cover, salt to taste, the wine, and the lemon juice. Bring the pot to a boil, uncovered.

4. Reduce heat and simmer uncovered for 5 minutes.

5. Turn off heat and leave the fish undisturbed for 10 minutes. Then remove carefully to a serving platter.

6. Serve fish warm or cold. Cold poached salmon is good with Green Garlic Dressing (see page 223).

Servings: 1 fillet per person. Calories 302, fat 6 g (24% of calories from fat), saturated fat 1 g, protein 35 g, carbohydrate 8 g, cholesterol 88 mg, fiber 2 g

Nutritional benefits: Good protein; omega-3 fatty acids

∽ *Salmon Cakes* ∾

4 ounces cooked salmon
2 tablespoons Green Garlic Dressing (see page 223)
¼ cup cooked corn kernels
2 teaspoons breadcrumbs
2 tablespoons yellow cornmeal (nondegerminated)
1 teaspoon light olive oil

1. Mash the fish and dressing together until smooth.
2. Fold in the corn kernels and breadcrumbs.
3. Form mixture into 2 patties, then press into the cornmeal to coat. Refrigerate for at least 1 hour before cooking.
4. Heat the olive oil in a small pan over high heat and cook patties for 1 or 2 minutes on each side to heat through.

Servings: 2. Calories 154, fat 6 g (30% of calories from fat), saturated fat 1 g, protein 13 g, carbohydrate 12 g, cholesterol 29 mg, fiber 1 g

Nutritional benefits: Protein, omega-3 fatty acids from salmon; protective phytochemicals

VEGETABLES

∽ *Oven-Fried Potatoes* ∾

3 medium, unpeeled baking potatoes (organic)
2 tablespoons fresh lemon juice
2 teaspoons extra-virgin olive oil
1½ teaspoons fresh rosemary, chopped fine (or 1 teaspoon dried rosemary, crumbled)
¼ teaspoon salt
¼ teaspoon freshly ground black pepper
2 cloves garlic, minced
vegetable cooking spray

1. Preheat oven to 400°F.
2. Wash and dry the potatoes and cut them in half lengthwise. Cut each half into 4 equal wedges.
3. Mix all the remaining ingredients (except the cooking spray) in a large bowl. Add the potatoes and toss well to coat.

4. Place the potatoes skin side down on a baking sheet coated with vegetable cooking spray. Do not crowd pieces.

5. Bake for 45 minutes or until tender and lightly browned.

Servings: 6. Calories 158, fat 2 g (9.5% of calories from fat), saturated fat less than 1 g, protein 4 g, carbohydrate 33 g, cholesterol 0 mg, sodium 100 mg, fiber 3 g

Nutritional benefits: Low in fat relative to standard French fries

∞ Oven-Roasted Vegetable Combo ∞

4–5 cups eggplant, cut in ¹/₂-inch dice
2 cups yams, peeled and cut in ¹/₂-inch dice
2 tablespoons extra-virgin olive oil
salt to taste

1. Preheat oven to 450°F.

2. Toss the vegetables in the olive oil and salt. Spread the vegetables in a single layer on a baking sheet.

3. Bake for 15 minutes, remove from oven, and flip as many pieces as you can with a spatula. (You don't have to flip every single piece.)

4. Bake for another 8 minutes.

Servings: 4. Calories 175, fat 7 g (35% of calories from fat), saturated fat 1 g, protein 2 g, carbohydrate 27 g, cholesterol 0 mg, fiber 6 g

Nutritional benefits: Micronutrients; monounsaturated fat

∞ Crusty Broiled Tomatoes ∞

2 ripe tomatoes
¹/₄ cup dried whole-grain breadcrumbs
1 tablespoon extra-virgin olive oil
1 clove garlic, minced
salt and black pepper to taste

1. Preheat oven to 350°F.

2. Halve the tomatoes horizontally and gently squeeze out loose seeds. Drain halves cut side down, then pat dry.

3. Combine the remaining ingredients and spoon mixture on cut sides of the tomatoes. Arrange the tomatoes in a baking dish.

4. Bake for 15 minutes, then place under the broiler just to brown the tops.

Servings: 2. Calories 117, fat 8 g (59% of calories from fat), saturated fat 1 g, protein 2 g, carbohydrate 10 g, cholesterol 0 mg, fiber less than 1 g

Nutritional benefits: Micronutrients; monounsaturated fat

∾ *Fragrant Spinach Purée* ∾

2 tablespoons raw cashew pieces
½ cup water
1 tablespoon extra-virgin olive oil
1 onion, sliced thin
1 tablespoon garlic, minced
1 tablespoon fresh gingerroot, peeled, grated, and minced
1 pound fresh spinach, cleaned and stemmed
1 tablespoon curry powder
salt to taste

1. Make nut milk: Grind cashew pieces in a blender until very fine, add the water, and blend for 2 minutes.

2. In a saucepan heat the olive oil over high heat. Add the onion and stir until it begins to brown.

2. Add the garlic and ginger, reduce heat to medium, and cook for a few minutes more.

3. Stir in the spinach and curry powder. Reduce heat to low and add the nut milk. Cover and simmer for 15 minutes.

4. Remove from heat, let cool slightly, then put mixture in a food processor and process until smooth.

5. Return the purée to saucepan, add salt to taste, and heat through.

Servings: 4. Calories 148, fat 4 g (23% of calories from fat), saturated fat 1.5 g, protein 10 g, carbohydrate 28.5 g, cholesterol 0 mg, fiber 7 g

Nutritional benefits: Micronutrients

෨෨ Sweet-and-Sour Stir-Fried Red Cabbage ෨෨

1 tablespoon extra-virgin olive oil
1 large onion, halved and sliced thin
6 cups finely shredded red cabbage
½ cup applesauce
¼ cup balsamic vinegar
2 tablespoons maple syrup
1 tablespoon caraway seeds
salt to taste

1. Heat the olive oil in a large skillet or wok. Add the onion and cook until browned. Add the cabbage, stir until well combined, and cook until the cabbage softens, about 3 minutes.

2. Meanwhile, combine the remaining ingredients in a small bowl. Add the mixture to the cabbage and continue stirring until heated through.

3. Add salt to taste. Serve warm or cold.

Servings: 4. Calories 103, fat 4 g (30% of calories from fat), saturated fat 0.5 g, protein 2 g, carbohydrate 18 g, cholesterol 0 mg, fiber 3 g
Nutritional benefits: Micronutrients; monounsaturated fat

෨෨ Green Cabbage and Mushrooms ෨෨

1 small green cabbage, cored and diced, about 6 cups
1 cup Vegetable Stock (see page 210)
1 tablespoon extra-virgin olive oil
1 medium onion, diced
½ pound mushrooms (shiitake or oyster, if possible)
1½ tablespoons cornstarch mixed into ¼ cup cold water
1 tablespoon fresh dill weed, chopped, or 1 teaspoon dried
½ teaspoon paprika
salt and black pepper to taste

1. In a covered pot over high heat, steam the cabbage in the stock for 5 minutes until it is just wilted and still bright green. Remove from heat and remove cover.

2. While the cabbage cooks, heat the olive oil in a large skillet or wok, and sauté the onion and mushrooms until they brown. Add the cabbage and heat through, mixing well. Stir the cornstarch mixture well and add it to skillet. Bring mixture to boil, stirring, until liquid thickens. Reduce heat and season to taste with dill, paprika, salt, and pepper.

Servings: 6. Calories 74, fat 3 g (36% of calories from fat), saturated fat 0.5 g, protein 2 g, carbohydrate 10 g, cholesterol 0 mg, fiber 1 g
Nutritional benefits: Micronutrients

PASTA, RICE, POTATOES

∽ *Pasta with Broccoli* ∽

1 large bunch broccoli
1 pound dried pasta (twists, penne, or rigatoni)
4 tablespoons extra-virgin olive oil
6 cloves garlic, minced
1 teaspoon red pepper flakes
salt to taste
2 tablespoons capers
1 cup freshly grated Parmesan cheese (optional)

1. Heat a large pot of water to cook the pasta.

2. Cut ½ inch off the ends of the broccoli stalks and cut the thick stalks away from the tops. Separate the tops into florets. Peel away the fibrous outer layer of the broccoli stalks and cut them into bite-size chunks.

3. Add the pasta to boiling water. While the pasta cooks, heat the olive oil in a small pan and add the garlic, red pepper, and salt to taste. Cook for 1–2 minutes, stirring, then remove from heat.

4. When the pasta is 2 minutes short of being *al dente,* add the broccoli. As soon as the broccoli is crunchy-tender (test a piece of stem), drain the broccoli-pasta mixture in a colander, return it to the pot, and add the oil mixture.

5. Add the capers, and season with salt to taste. Serve with the grated Parmesan cheese, if desired.

Servings: 6. Calories 431, fat 14 g (30% of calories from fat), saturated fat 4 g, protein 16 g, carbohydrate 59 g, cholesterol 10 mg, fiber 2 g

Nutritional benefits: Good carbohydrate; micronutrients from broccoli; monounsaturated fat

∽ *Chinese Noodles with Broccoli* ∾

1 pound broccoli
1 pound dried pasta (linguine or fettucine)
2 tablespoons dark (roasted) sesame oil
1 tablespoon light olive oil
2 tablespoons garlic, minced
1 teaspoon hot red pepper flakes
1 package (6 ounces) baked, pressed tofu, cut into ½-inch cubes
6 tablespoons reduced-sodium soy sauce
3 tablespoons rice wine vinegar
2 tablespoons light brown sugar

1. Cut ½ inch off the ends of the broccoli stalks and cut the thick stalks away from the tops. Separate the tops into florets. Peel away the fibrous outer layer of the broccoli stalks and cut them into bite-size chunks.

2. Bring a large pot of water to the boil. Add the broccoli and cook until crunchy-tender, about 4–5 minutes. Remove the broccoli with a slotted spoon and rinse it under cold water. Drain.

3. Add the pasta to the boiling water and cook it until it is *al dente*.

4. While the pasta is cooking, heat the sesame oil and olive oil in a skillet. Add the garlic and red pepper and stir-fry for 10 seconds. Add the broccoli, tofu cubes, soy sauce, vinegar, and brown sugar, and stir-fry for 30 seconds. Remove from heat.

5. Drain the pasta and toss it with the broccoli mixture. Serve warm or at room temperature.

Servings: 6. Calories 429, fat 11 g (23% of calories from fat), saturated fat 1.6 g, protein 17.4 g, carbohydrate 64 g, cholesterol 0 mg, sodium 724 mg, fiber 2 g

Nutritional benefits: Good carbohydrate; protein, calcium, and isoflavones from tofu; micronutrients from broccoli and garlic

∽ Pasta with Winter Squash and Walnuts ∾

1 pound winter squash, such as buttercup, kabocha, or banana,
peeled, seeded, and cubed
1 pound dried pasta, such as bowties or shells
1 tablespoon extra-virgin olive oil
2 cloves garlic, minced
3 tablespoons fresh parsley, minced
salt and black or red pepper to taste
2 tablespoons walnuts, chopped
1/4 cup Parmesan cheese, grated

1. Place the squash in a saucepan with a little water, cover, and steam until it is soft. Drain and mash the squash.

2. Cook the pasta until it is *al dente*.

3. While the pasta is cooking, heat the olive oil in a skillet, add the garlic, and sauté for 30 seconds. Add the mashed squash, the parsley, and salt and pepper to taste.

4. Toss the drained pasta with the squash mixture and serve topped with the chopped walnuts and grated Parmesan cheese.

Servings: 6. Calories 361, fat 6 g (15% of calories from fat), saturated fat 1.2 g, protein 13 g, carbohydrate 64 g, cholesterol 3 mg, fiber 3 g
Nutritional benefits: Good carbohydrate; omega-3 fatty acids from walnuts; micronutrients from winter squash, garlic, and parsley

∽ Pasta Puttanesca ∾

5–6 cups fresh tomatoes, peeled, seeded, and crushed (or use canned Italian
tomatoes, drained and crushed)
1 tablespoon extra-virgin olive oil
1 teaspoon dried hot red pepper flakes
1 1/2 tablespoons capers, drained and rinsed
3 tablespoons black olives (Kalamata or oil-cured), pitted and chopped
1 tablespoon garlic, minced
2 tablespoons fresh basil leaves, minced
1 pound dried penne pasta
3/4 cup Parmesan cheese, grated

1. In a large bowl, combine the tomatoes, olive oil, red pepper flakes, capers, olives, garlic, and basil. Let stand at room temperature for 1 hour.

2. Cook the pasta until it is *al dente*. Drain well.

3. Toss the hot pasta with the tomato mixture. Add the grated Parmesan cheese and serve immediately.

Servings: 6. Calories 391, fat 7.5 g (17% of calories from fat), saturated fat 2.5 g, protein 15.5 g, carbohydrate 66 g, cholesterol 8 mg, sodium 247 mg, fiber 4 g

Nutritional benefits: Good carbohydrate; micronutrients from tomatoes and garlic

🍝 Pasta with Kale 🍝

½ cup sun-dried tomatoes
1 pound dried pasta (penne, rigatoni, or twists)
2 tablespoons extra-virgin olive oil
1 large onion, thinly sliced
½ teaspoon hot red pepper flakes
1 pound kale, coarse stems and midribs removed, coarsely chopped
4 cloves garlic, minced
2 tablespoons capers with 1 tablespoon of their juice
salt to taste
¾ cup freshly grated Parmesan cheese (optional)

1. Soak the sun-dried tomatoes in hot water until they are soft, about 10 minutes. Drain, cut them into pieces, and reserve.

2. Begin cooking the pasta. While the pasta is cooking, heat the olive oil in a large skillet and sauté the onion over medium-high heat until it is golden. Add the red pepper flakes and the sun-dried tomatoes, and stir-fry for 1 minute more.

3. Add the kale, tossing well to wilt. Add the garlic and cook, stirring frequently for 5 minutes. Add the capers and their juice and remove from heat.

4. When the pasta is cooked *al dente,* remove from heat, drain well, and mix it with the kale. Add salt to taste. Serve with the grated Parmesan cheese, if desired.

Servings: 6. Calories 550, fat 9 g (15% of calories from fat), saturated fat 1 g, protein 19.5 g, carbohydrate 99 g, cholesterol 0 mg, fiber 7 g

Nutritional benefits: Good carbohydrate; micronutrients from kale; monounsaturated fat

Marinara Sauce for Pasta

> 2 tablespoons extra-virgin olive oil
> 2 medium onions, chopped
> 1 medium carrot, peeled and finely grated
> 1 teaspoon salt
> 1/4 teaspoon red pepper flakes, or to taste
> 1 large can (28 ounces) Italian tomatoes, crushed
> 1 large can (16 ounces) tomato paste
> 1 teaspoon sugar (optional)
> 1 bay leaf (Turkish)
> 2 tablespoons dried whole basil
> 1 teaspoon dried whole oregano
> scant pinch fennel seeds
> 1/4 teaspoon ground allspice
> 4 cloves garlic, mashed
> salt to taste

1. Heat the olive oil in a large pot (do not use cast iron or aluminum) over medium-high heat. Add the onions and carrot and sauté until the onions are translucent.

2. Add the salt and red pepper flakes, then the tomatoes and tomato paste. Mix well, bring just to a boil, lower heat, and continue to cook at a simmer.

3. Add the sugar, herbs, and spices, and simmer uncovered for 30 minutes, stirring occasionally.

4. Add the garlic, and continue to simmer for 30 minutes more or until desired thickness. Add salt to taste. Remove the bay leaf.

Servings: 8. Calories 73, fat 4 g (43% of calories from fat), saturated fat 0.5 g, protein 1.5 g, carbohydrate 10 g, cholesterol 0 mg, sodium 402 mg, fiber 2 g

Nutritional benefits: Multiple micronutrients, including lycopene from tomatoes; monounsaturated fat

৩৩ Stir-Fried Rice ৩৩

1 tablespoon light olive oil
1 small onion or 3 scallions, chopped
2 cloves garlic, minced
1 tablespoon fresh gingerroot, peeled, grated, and minced
1 package (6 ounces) baked, pressed tofu, diced
4 cups cooked, cooled rice
3 tablespoons reduced-sodium soy sauce
½ cup cooked peas
2 tablespoons coriander (cilantro) leaves, chopped
1 teaspoon dark (roasted) sesame oil

1. In a wok or large skillet, heat the olive oil, and quickly sauté the onion, garlic, and ginger, stirring constantly with a large spoon.

2. Add the tofu and warm it through.

3. Add the rice, stirring and turning it to mix it with the other ingredients and warm it through. Add the soy sauce and mix well.

4. Add the peas, coriander, and sesame oil, and mix well.

Servings: 6. Calories 698, fat 9 g (11% of calories from fat), saturated fat 1 g, protein 19 g, carbohydrate 136 g, cholesterol 0 mg, sodium 897 mg, fiber 5 g

Nutritional benefits: Micronutrients; protein, calcium, and isoflavones from tofu

৩৩ Porcini Risotto ৩৩

¼ cup dried porcini mushrooms
3–4 cups warm Vegetable Stock (see page 210)
1 tablespoon extra-virgin olive oil
1 small onion, minced
1 cup Arborio rice
salt and pepper to taste
2 teaspoons truffle-flavored olive oil (optional)
¼ cup grated fresh Parmesan cheese (optional)

1. Rinse the dried mushrooms in cold water, drain, and add to warm vegetable stock to soften.

2. In a large skillet, heat the olive oil over medium heat and sauté the onion until soft. Add the rice and stir to combine. Add the mushrooms, cut into smaller pieces if necessary. Reduce heat to medium-low.

3. Add the stock, one ladleful at a time, as you stir the rice. As the rice absorbs the liquid, add more. After 15 minutes, test the rice for doneness.

4. When the rice is tender but not mushy, remove from heat, season to taste with salt and pepper, and add truffle-flavored olive oil and grated Parmesan cheese, if desired.

Servings: 4. Calories 411, fat 9 g (19.5% of calories from fat), saturated fat 2 g, protein 12 g, carbohydrate 70 g, cholesterol 6 mg, fiber 2.5 g

Nutritional benefits: Medium-glycemic-index carbohydrate; monounsaturated fat; micronutrients

⟢ Stuffed Green Potatoes ⟣

3 large baking potatoes
3 stalks broccoli
½ teaspoon salt
1 tablespoon extra-virgin olive oil
2 tablespoons soy milk
2 tablespoons Parmesan cheese, grated

1. Preheat oven to 400°F. Scrub the potatoes and make shallow cuts around their middles to make it easier to cut them in half lengthwise after baking. Bake the potatoes until soft, about 1 hour, depending on their size.

2. Meanwhile, cut the ends from the stalks of broccoli and peel some of the outer skin off to make the stems more edible. Steam the broccoli until it is crunchy-tender and bright green, about 5 minutes. Drain and chop fine.

3. Cut the potatoes in half and scoop out the insides into a bowl. Add the salt, olive oil, and soy milk, and mash the potatoes into a smooth paste. Add the grated Parmesan cheese and the chopped broccoli and mix well.

4. Pile the mixture back into the potato shells, arrange on a baking dish, and heat them through. (Kids love these.)

Servings: 6. Calories 101, fat 3 g (26% of calories from fat), saturated fat less than 1 g, protein 4 g, carbohydrate 16 g, cholesterol 1 mg, sodium 226 mg, fiber 3 g

Nutritional benefits: Micronutrients

✌ Couscous ✌

1½ cups boiling water
⅔ cup whole-wheat couscous
1 teaspoon extra-virgin olive oil
1 fresh Italian tomato, chopped
1 tablespoon fresh parsley leaves, chopped
1 clove garlic, minced
salt to taste
1 tablespoon capers
2 tablespoons slivered almonds, toasted

1. Pour boiling water over the couscous in a mixing bowl. Stir, cover, and let stand for 10 minutes.

2. Loosen the grains with a fork, stir in the olive oil, then add the other ingredients. Add salt to taste.

3. Serve at room temperature.

Servings: 4. Calories 147, fat 3 g (20% of calories from fat), saturated fat less than 1 g, protein 5 g, carbohydrate 25 g, cholesterol 0 mg, fiber 2 g

Nutritional benefits: Whole-grain carbohydrate; micronutrients

DESSERTS

✌ Banana Bread ✌

4–5 very ripe bananas
¾ cup honey, liquefied in microwave (30 seconds)
¼ cup light olive oil
2 teaspoons vanilla extract
2 cups whole-wheat pastry flour, sifted
2 teaspoons baking soda
¾ cup walnuts, chopped

1. Preheat oven to 350°F.

2. Mash the bananas thoroughly and mix well with the honey, olive oil, and vanilla extract.

3. Mix separately the sifted flour, baking soda, and walnuts.

4. Blend the dry ingredients into the wet ones, stirring until just mixed.

5. Put the batter into a nonstick 8-inch-square baking pan and bake for 45–60 minutes until a knife inserted in the center comes out clean. Remove from oven, let cool slightly, and remove from pan.

Servings: 9. Calories 339, fat 12.5 g (31% of calories from fat), saturated fat 1.5 g, protein 7 g, carbohydrate 56 g, cholesterol 0 mg, sodium 283 mg, fiber 5 g

Nutritional benefits: Monounsaturated fat; omega-3 fatty acids from walnuts; micronutrients

℘ Carrot Cake ℘

2 cups (firmly packed) peeled, finely grated carrots
juice of 1 large orange
2 teaspoons vanilla extract
¼ cup light olive oil
1 cup honey, liquefied in microwave (30 seconds)
½ cup crushed or chopped pineapple
1 cup unbleached white flour
1½ cups whole-wheat pastry flour
2 teaspoons baking soda
1 teaspoon cinnamon
½ teaspoon ground allspice
¾ cup walnuts, chopped

1. Preheat oven to 350°F.

2. Mix together the carrots, orange juice, vanilla, olive oil, honey, and pineapple.

3. Sift together the flours, baking soda, and spices. Mix in the walnuts.

4. Blend the dry ingredients into the wet ones, stirring until just mixed.

5. Put the batter into a nonstick 8-inch-square baking pan and bake for 45–60 minutes until a knife inserted in the center comes out clean. Remove from oven, let cool slightly, and remove from pan.

Servings: 9. Calories 375, fat 12.5 g (29% of calories from fat), saturated fat 1 g, protein 7 g, carbohydrate 63 g, cholesterol 0 mg, sodium 291 mg, fiber 5 g

Nutritional benefits: Monounsaturated fat; omega-3 fatty acids from walnuts; micronutrients

∞ *Apple Crisp* ∞

12 large green apples, peeled, cored, and sliced
juice of 1 fresh lemon
¼ cup raisins
⅓ cup brandy
¼ cup light brown sugar, packed
1 teaspoon cinnamon
2 tablespoons whole-wheat pastry flour
1½ cups old-fashioned rolled oats
½ cup toasted wheat germ
¾ teaspoon salt
1½ teaspoons cinnamon
½ cup brown sugar, packed
⅓ cup light olive oil
⅓ cup maple syrup
nonstick cooking spray

1. Preheat oven to 375°F.
2. In a mixing bowl, toss the apples with the lemon juice, raisins, brandy, brown sugar, 1 teaspoon cinnamon, and the flour.
3. Pile the apples in a glass or ceramic baking dish sprayed with nonstick cooking spray.
4. Mix together the remaining ingredients and cover the apples with the mixture.

5. Cover the baking dish with aluminum foil and bake 20 minutes. Uncover and bake 30–40 minutes more until the apples are soft. Serve warm.

Servings: 12. Calories 244, fat 7.5 g (27.5% of calories from fat), saturated fat 1 g, protein 4 g, carbohydrate 40 g, cholesterol 0 mg, sodium 140 mg, fiber 5 g

Nutritional benefits: Fiber and carbohydrate from whole grains; monounsaturated fat; micronutrients

✇ Tart Cherry-Apple Crunch ✇

1 pound frozen pitted dark cherries
1 green apple, cored and diced
¼ cup light brown sugar, packed
½ teaspoon almond extract
1½ tablespoons arrowroot powder
½ cup unsweetened cherry or apple juice
nonstick cooking spray
¼ cup old-fashioned rolled oats
¼ cup brown sugar
¼ cup walnuts, chopped
2 tablespoons whole-wheat pastry flour
3 tablespoons light olive oil
¼ teaspoon salt (optional)

1. Preheat oven to 400°F.

2. In a bowl, toss together the cherries, apple, brown sugar, and almond extract.

3. In a cup, mix the arrowroot and juice well and add to the fruit mixture, stirring well.

4. Pour the mixture into an 8-inch-square baking dish sprayed with nonstick cooking spray.

5. Mix together the remaining ingredients and put the mixture on top of the fruit.

6. Bake for 30 minutes. Raise heat to broil and brown topping lightly for 1–2 minutes. Remove from oven. Serve warm or cold.

Servings: 6. Calories 281, fat 10 g (31.5% of calories from fat), saturated fat 1 g, protein 2 g, carbohydrate 48 g, cholesterol 0 mg, sodium 9 mg, fiber 4 g

Nutritional benefits: Micronutrients; monounsaturated fat; omega-3 fatty acids from walnuts

✺ Pumpkin Muffins ✺

2 cups pumpkin purée
³/₄–1 cup maple syrup (depending on sweetness of pumpkin)
3 tablespoons light olive oil
2 cups whole-wheat pastry flour
1 teaspoon baking soda
¹/₂ teaspoon salt (optional)
¹/₄ teaspoon ground cloves
¹/₄ teaspoon powdered ginger
1 teaspoon cinnamon
³/₄ cup walnuts, chopped

1. Preheat oven to 350°F.

2. Mix together the pumpkin purée, maple syrup, and olive oil.

3. Sift together the flour, baking soda, salt (if desired), and spices, and add the walnuts.

4. Blend the dry ingredients into the wet ones until just mixed.

5. Divide the batter equally in the 12 cups of a nonstick muffin pan.

6. Bake for 45 minutes. Remove from oven, let cool slightly, and remove muffins from pan.

Servings: 12. Calories 211, fat 8.5 g (33.5% of calories from fat), saturated fat 1 g, protein 5 g, carbohydrate 32 g, cholesterol 0 mg, sodium 199 mg, fiber 4 g

Nutritional benefits: Micronutrients; omega-3 fatty acids from walnuts; monounsaturated fat

∞ Easy Pie Crust ∞

1 package (1/3 pound) natural Graham crackers
2 1/2 tablespoons maple syrup
2 tablespoons sesame tahini
1 1/2 teaspoons water

1. Pulverize the Graham crackers in a food processor.
2. Add the remaining ingredients and process until well blended.
3. Press mixture evenly into a 9-inch pie pan.
4. If an unbaked filling is to be used, bake the crust in an oven heated to 350°F for 20–30 minutes until lightly browned. Otherwise, add the filling and bake the pie as directed.

Servings: 8. Calories 355, fat 4 g (10% of calories from fat), saturated fat 1 g, protein 2.7 g, carbohydrate 81 g, cholesterol 0 mg, sodium 137 mg, fiber 1 g

Nutritional benefits: Micronutrients; little saturated fat

∞ Fruit "Pizza" ∞

mixture for 1 Easy Pie Crust (see above)
1 pound firm tofu
1 teaspoon vanilla extract
finely grated zest of 2 lemons (organic)
1/4 cup sugar
2 cups fresh fruit (blueberries, sliced strawberries, peaches, kiwis, grapes)
1/4 cup orange marmalade
1 teaspoon fresh lemon juice

1. Preheat oven to 350°F.
2. Press the crust mixture into a 14-inch pizza pan and bake for 20 minutes. Remove from heat, cool, and place in the freezer to chill.
3. Drain the tofu and process in a food processor until smooth, adding the vanilla extract, lemon zest, and sugar.
4. Spread the mixture on top of the chilled crust and refrigerate for at least 1 hour.
5. Arrange the sliced fruit on top of the tofu mixture.

6. In a small glass or ceramic bowl, heat the marmalade and lemon juice in a microwave until bubbly. Drizzle the mixture over the pizza and chill 1 hour more.

Servings: 8. Calories 467, fat 7 g (13.5% of calories from fat), saturated fat 1 g, protein 7.5 g, carbohydrate 99 g, cholesterol 0 mg, sodium 148 mg, fiber 3 g

Nutritional benefits: Protein, calcium, and isoflavones from tofu; micronutrients; little saturated fat

❧ *Holiday Squash Pie* ❧

½ cup raw cashew pieces
1 cup water
4½ tablespoons arrowroot powder
6 cups cooked puréed winter squash (buttercup, banana, or hubbard)
½ cup sugar
½ cup light brown sugar, packed
4 tablespoons brandy
¾ teaspoon powdered ginger
⅜ teaspoon ground cloves
1½ teaspoons cinnamon
¾ cup walnuts, chopped
2 unbaked Easy Pie Crusts (see page 250)

1. Preheat oven to 400°F.

2. In a blender, grind the cashew pieces until very fine. Add the water and blend on high speed for 2 minutes. Add the arrowroot powder and blend on low speed for 30 seconds. Keep the mixture in the blender until needed.

3. In a food processor or mixer combine the squash purée, sugars, brandy, and spices.

4. Blend the cashew/arrowroot mixture for another few seconds, then add to the squash mixture and process until well mixed.

5. Divide the pie filling equally between the two pie crusts. Top with the chopped walnuts. Bake the pies for 50–60 minutes until lightly browned, cracked, and well set.

6. Remove the pies from the oven, cool, then refrigerate overnight to allow filling to firm up. Serve cool or at room temperature.

Servings: 16 (8 per pie). Calories 491, fat 9.5 g (17.5% of calories from fat), saturated fat 1.5 g, protein 5.5 g, carbohydrate 100 g, cholesterol 0 mg, sodium 142 mg, fiber 3 g

Nutritional benefits: Micronutrients; omega-3 fatty acids from walnuts; no saturated fat

ஒ   *Raspberry Chocolate Pie*   ஒ

> mixture for 1 Easy Pie Crust (see page 250)
> 3 tablespoons unsweetened cocoa powder
> 1 tablespoon maple syrup
> 1½ pounds frozen raspberries, thawed and drained (liquid reserved)
> 2 tablespoons arrowroot powder
> ½ cup light brown sugar
> 1 teaspoon almond extract

1. Preheat oven to 350°F.
2. To the Easy Pie Crust mixture, add the cocoa and maple syrup and process in a food processor until well blended. Press the mixture into a 9-inch pie pan and bake for 20 minutes until lightly browned. Cool.
3. Combine the reserved raspberry liquid and the arrowroot in a saucepan until smooth. Add the brown sugar and gently fold in the berries. Place over medium heat and stir with a wooden spoon until mixture becomes clear and thickens. Cook for 1 minute more. Add the almond extract. Cool.
4. Spoon the raspberry mixture into pie crust. Refrigerate at least 2 hours before serving.

Servings: 8. Calories 513, fat 4.5 g (8% of calories from fat), saturated fat 1 g, protein 4 g, carbohydrate 121 g, cholesterol 0 mg, sodium 144 mg, fiber 5.5 g

Nutritional benefits: Micronutrients, including high fiber from raspberries

✎ Blueberry Cream Pie ✎

1 pound silken tofu
¼ cup sugar, or more to taste
2 teaspoons vanilla extract
finely grated zest of 1 fresh lemon (organic)
1 baked Easy Pie Crust (see page 250)
1 pound fresh or frozen blueberries
¼ cup light brown sugar
1 tablespoon fresh lemon juice
½ teaspoon cinnamon
1½ tablespoons arrowroot powder
2 tablespoons cold water

1. Drain the tofu well and process in a food processor until smooth. Add the sugar, vanilla extract, and lemon zest, and blend well.

2. Pour the tofu mixture into the pie crust and chill in refrigerator.

3. Place the blueberries in a saucepan and cook over medium heat until they begin to boil. Boil gently for 10 minutes.

4. Add the brown sugar, lemon juice, and cinnamon, and cook for another 2 minutes.

5. Mix the arrowroot well with the water, and pour mixture into the simmering blueberries while stirring. Cook, stirring, until the mixture becomes clear and thick. Continue to cook for 1 minute. Remove from heat and cool.

6. When blueberry mixture is cool, spoon it over the tofu mixture, and refrigerate the pie for 2 hours before serving.

Servings: 8. Calories 430, fat 7 g (15% of calories from fat), saturated fat 1.5 g, protein 7 g, carbohydrate 90 g, cholesterol 0 mg, sodium 141 mg, fiber 2 g

Nutritional benefits: Protein, calcium, and isoflavones from tofu; low-glycemic-index carbohydrate and micronutrients from blueberries

∞ *Blueberry Pie* ∞

1½ pounds fresh or frozen blueberries
½ cup light brown sugar
juice of ½ fresh lemon
1 teaspoon cinnamon
2 tablespoons arrowroot powder
2 tablespoons cold water
1 baked Easy Pie Crust (see page 250)

1. Heat the blueberries in a saucepan over medium heat until they begin to boil. Boil gently for 10 minutes.

2. Add the brown sugar, lemon juice, and cinnamon, and cook for another 2 minutes.

3. Mix the arrowroot well with the water, and pour mixture into the simmering blueberries while stirring. Cook, stirring, until mixture becomes clear and thick. Continue to cook for 1 minute. Remove from heat and cool.

4. Spoon mixture into the pie crust and refrigerate for at least 2 hours before serving.

Servings: 8. Calories 461, fat 3 g (6% of calories from fat), saturated fat 1 g, protein 3 g, carbohydrate 108 g, cholesterol 0 mg, sodium 144 mg, fiber 4 g

Nutritional benefits: Low-glycemic-index carbohydrate from blueberries; micronutrients

∞ *Frozen Banana Pie* ∞

6 very ripe bananas, peeled
¼ cup natural or light brown sugar
1 tablespoon fresh lime juice
1 teaspoon cinnamon
1 teaspoon vanilla extract
1 baked Easy Pie Crust (see page 250)
1–2 cups fresh berries or other fruit, sliced

1. Place all the ingredients except the pie crust and berries in a blender or food processor and process until smooth.

2. Pour the mixture in the pie crust, and freeze the pie solid.

3. Remove the pie 15 minutes before serving and cover the top with the fruit.

Servings: 8. Calories 462, fat 3 g (6.5% of calories from fat), saturated fat 1 g, protein 3.5 g, carbohydrate 108 g, cholesterol 0 mg, sodium 141 mg, fiber 2.5 g

Nutritional benefits: Micronutrients; little saturated fat

∽ *Carrot-Nut Torte* ∽

1 pound carrots, peeled and grated (about 3½ cups)
1 tablespoon fresh gingerroot, peeled, grated, and finely chopped
1 cup walnuts, coarsely ground
½ cup light brown sugar, packed
½ cup maple syrup
¼ cup light olive oil
1 teaspoon vanilla extract
1 teaspoon almond extract
2 tablespoons rum
¾ cup whole-wheat pastry flour
¼ cup unbleached white flour
1 tablespoon baking powder
nonstick cooking spray

1. Preheat the oven to 350°F.

2. Combine the carrots, ginger, walnuts, brown sugar, maple syrup, olive oil, extracts, and rum.

3. In a separate bowl, sift together the flours and baking powder.

4. Fold the dry ingredients into the wet ones. Put the batter into a 9-inch spring-form pan coated with nonstick cooking spray.

5. Bake for 60 minutes, remove from oven, and allow to cool before slicing.

Servings: 8. Calories 326, fat 18 g (42.5% of calories from fat), saturated fat 1.5 g, protein 6 g, carbohydrate 43 g, cholesterol 0 mg, sodium 162 mg, fiber 4 g

Nutritional benefits: Monounsaturated fat; omega-3 fatty acids from walnuts

෨෨   Chocolate Tapioca Pudding   ෨෨

¹/₂ cup medium pearl tapioca
4 cups vanilla-flavored soy milk
¹/₄ cup unsweetened cocoa powder
¹/₂ cup light brown sugar
2 teaspoons vanilla extract

1. Soak the tapioca overnight in cold water to cover. Drain.
2. Combine the tapioca with the soy milk, cocoa, and sugar in a saucepan.
3. Place the tapioca over medium heat and boil gently, stirring frequently until the mixture thickens and the pearls look clear, about 45 minutes. Remove from heat and stir in the vanilla extract.
4. Serve warm or cold.

Servings: 4. Calories 178, fat 3.5 g (17% of calories from fat), saturated fat 0.5 g, protein 5 g, carbohydrate 34.5 g, cholesterol 0 mg, sodium 27 mg, fiber 3.5 g

Nutritional benefits: Isoflavones from soy milk; little saturated fat

෨෨   Indian Pudding   ෨෨

4 cups vanilla-flavored soy milk
¹/₂ cup plus 2 tablespoons yellow cornmeal (nondegerminated)
¹/₂ cup brown sugar
¹/₄ cup unsulfured molasses or maple syrup
¹/₂ teaspoon powdered ginger
1 teaspoon cinnamon
¹/₄ teaspoon ground cloves
¹/₄ teaspoon salt

1. Preheat oven to 300°F.
2. In a medium saucepan over high heat, bring the soy milk to a boil. Reduce heat to low and sprinkle in the cornmeal while stirring. Add the remaining ingredients and simmer 15 minutes, stirring occasionally. Remove from heat and pour into a lightly oiled ovenproof dish.

3. Bake the pudding 45–60 minutes until browned and set. Remove from oven. Serve warm.

Servings: 6. Calories 213, fat 3.5 g (14% of calories from fat), saturated fat 0.5 g, protein 6 g, carbohydrate 42 g, cholesterol 0 mg, sodium 121 mg, fiber 3 g

Nutritional benefits: Isoflavones from soy milk

∽ Oatmeal Cookies ∾

³/₄ cup whole-wheat pastry flour
³/₄ cup unbleached white flour
1 teaspoon baking powder
¹/₈ teaspoon salt (optional)
1 teaspoon cinnamon
¹/₄ teaspoon ground nutmeg
1¹/₂ cups old-fashioned rolled oats
1 cup any combination of chopped walnuts, raisins, and dates
6 ounces silken tofu
¹/₂ cup light olive oil
¹/₄ cup water
1 cup light brown sugar, packed
2 tablespoons vanilla extract

1. Preheat oven to 375°F.

2. Sift together the flours, baking powder, salt, and spices. Stir in the oats and the fruit/nut mix.

3. In a separate bowl, mash the tofu with the back of a fork or wooden spoon and stir in the remaining ingredients.

4. Using a rubber spatula, fold the wet ingredients into the dry ones, combining thoroughly.

5. Drop the batter by tablespoons on an ungreased cookie sheet and press each down slightly with a fork. Bake the cookies about 10 minutes or until the edges just begin to brown.

Servings: 48. Calories 78, fat 3.5 g (39% of calories from fat), saturated fat 0.5 g, protein 1 g, carbohydrate 11 g, cholesterol 0 mg, sodium 8 mg, fiber 1 g

Nutritional benefits: Almost no saturated fat

∽ Sesame-Almond Cookies ∽

3/4 cup whole-wheat pastry flour
3/4 cup unbleached white flour
1 teaspoon baking powder
1/8 teaspoon salt (optional)
1/4 cup sesame seeds, toasted
3/4 cup raw almonds, coarsely chopped
4 ounces silken tofu, drained
1/2 cup light olive oil
3/4 cup light brown sugar, packed
1 tablespoon almond extract

1. Preheat oven to 350°F.

2. In a bowl, sift together the flours, baking powder, and salt (if desired). Mix in the sesame seeds and chopped almonds.

3. In another bowl, mash the tofu and combine with the olive oil, brown sugar, and almond extract.

4. Using a rubber spatula, fold the wet ingredients into the dry ones. Roll the mixture into 1-inch balls, flatten between your palms, and place them on ungreased baking sheets. Bake the cookies about 10 minutes, until the edges begin to brown.

Servings: 48. Calories 88, fat 5 g (52% of calories from fat), saturated fat 1 g, protein 1.5 g, carbohydrate 9 g, cholesterol 0 mg, sodium 45 mg, fiber 1 g

Nutritional benefits: Protein, calcium, and isoflavones from tofu; calcium and fiber from sesame seeds; little saturated fat

∽ Almond-Butter Cookies ∽

3/4 cup whole-wheat pastry flour
3/4 cup unbleached white flour
1 teaspoon baking powder
1/8 teaspoon salt (optional)
4 ounces silken tofu, drained
1/4 cup plus 2 tablespoons chunky almond butter
1/4 cup plus 2 tablespoons light olive oil
1/2 cup light brown sugar, packed

¹/₄ cup maple syrup
1 tablespoon vanilla extract

1. Preheat oven to 350°F.

2. In a bowl, sift together the flours, baking powder, and salt (if desired).

3. In another bowl, mash the tofu and combine with the almond butter, olive oil, brown sugar, maple syrup, and vanilla extract.

4. Using a rubber spatula, fold the wet ingredients into the dry ones. Roll the mixture into 1-inch balls, place on ungreased baking sheets, and press flat with the back of a fork. Bake the cookies about 10 minutes until the edges just begin to brown.

Servings: 48. Calories 42, fat 1 g (28% of calories from fat), saturated fat 0 g, protein 1 g, carbohydrate 7 g, cholesterol 0 mg, sodium 15 mg, fiber 0.5 g

Nutritional benefits: Protein, calcium, and isoflavones from tofu; no saturated fat

∽ Walnut Cookies ∽

³/₄ cup whole-wheat pastry flour
³/₄ cup unbleached white flour
1 teaspoon baking powder
¹/₈ teaspoon salt (optional)
¹/₂ cup walnuts, chopped
4 ounces silken tofu
¹/₂ cup light olive oil
¹/₂ cup light brown sugar, packed
¹/₄ cup maple syrup
1 tablespoon vanilla extract

1. Preheat oven to 350°F.

2. In a bowl, sift together the flours, baking powder, and salt (if desired). Mix in the walnuts.

3. In another bowl, mash the tofu and combine with the olive oil, brown sugar, maple syrup, and vanilla extract.

4. Using a rubber spatula, fold the wet ingredients into the dry ones. Drop the batter by rounded teaspoonfuls onto ungreased

baking sheets and bake the cookies for 10–12 minutes until the edges just begin to brown.

Servings: 48. Calories 50, fat 3 g (55% of calories from fat), saturated fat 0.5 g, protein 1 g, carbohydrate 5 g, cholesterol 0 mg, sodium 14 mg, fiber 0.5 g

Nutritional benefits: Omega-3 fatty acids in walnuts; little saturated fat

APPENDIX A

THE OPTIMUM DIET

Throughout this book I have made references to "the optimum diet." Here I want to summarize its characteristics. The optimum diet should:

- supply all of your needs for calories, macronutrients, and micronutrients
- support general health throughout life and maximize longevity
- provide the pleasure you expect from eating
- promote social interaction and reinforce your personal and cultural identity

GENERAL CHARACTERISTICS OF THE OPTIMUM DIET

- *Variety.* Covering all nutritional bases and minimizing the intake of any harmful elements in foods are important.
- *Freshness.* The higher the percentage of fresh foods in the diet the better.
- *Unprocessed.* The lower the percentage of processed foods in the diet the better.
- *Abundant in fruits and vegetables.* The more fruits and vegetables you eat, the more protective phytochemicals you take in.

CALORIES

Depending on gender, body size, and activity level, most adults need to consume between 2,000 and 3,000 calories a day. Women, and smaller and less active people, need fewer calories; men, and bigger and more active people, need more. If you are eating the appropriate number of calories and not varying your activity, your weight should not fluctuate greatly.

Distribution of calories should be as follows: 50 to 60 percent from carbohydrates, 30 percent from fat, and 10 to 20 percent from protein.

CARBOHYDRATES

Adult women should eat about 225 to 270 grams of carbohydrates a day, while men should eat about 288 to 345 grams. The majority of this should be in the form of less-refined, less-processed foods with a low (i.e., below 60) glycemic index, and you should try to eat some low-GI carbohydrate food with each meal (whole grains, beans, vegetables, and nontropical fruits). If you eat high-GI carbohydrates, try to include them in mixed meals that contain some low-GI foods.

Try to reduce consumption of foods made with wheat flour and sugar and increase consumption of legumes.

FAT

On a 2,000-calorie-a-day diet, 600 calories can come from fat—that is, about 67 grams. This should be in a ratio of 1:2:1 of saturated to monounsaturated to polyunsaturated fat, meaning that no more than 100 calories should come from saturated fat. Reduce saturated fat by eating less butter, cream, cheese, and other full-fat dairy products, unskinned chicken, fatty meats, and products made with palm and coconut oil. The polyunsaturated fat in your diet should have a ratio of omega-6 to omega-3 fatty acids in the range of 2–4 to 1. In practice, this means reducing consumption of polyunsaturated vegetable oils and increasing consumption of oily fish, fortified eggs, soybeans, walnuts, or hemp or flax seeds.

Avoid margarine, vegetable shortening, all products made with partially hydrogenated oils, and fried foods in restaurants, especially fast-food restaurants.

PROTEIN

Daily intake should be between 50 and 100 grams on a 2,000-calorie-a-day diet. Eat less protein if you have liver or kidney problems, allergies, or autoimmunity problem. Eat more vegetable protein, especially from beans, in general, and soybeans, in particular, and less animal protein, except for fish and reduced-fat dairy products. Avoid protein supplements.

Vitamins and Minerals

Eating a diet high in fresh foods with plenty of fruits and vegetables will provide most of the micronutrients you need. In addition, I recommend supplementing the diet with the following:

- vitamin C, 100 mg twice a day
- vitamin E, 400 to 800 IU of a natural form (d-alpha-tocopherol together with other tocopherols)
- selenium, 200 mcg of a yeast-bound form
- mixed carotenoids, 25,000 IU
- a B-complex vitamin providing at least 400 mcg of folic acid
- calcium, 1,200 to 1,500 mg as calcium carbonate (for those under sixty-five) or calcium citrate (for those sixty-five and over).

Fiber

The optimum diet should provide 40 grams of fiber a day. You can achieve this by increasing consumption of fruits (especially berries), vegetables (especially beans), and whole grains.

Protective Phytochemicals

To get maximum natural protection against cancer, degenerative disease, and environmental toxicity, eat a variety of fruits, vegetables, and mushrooms, and drink tea, especially green tea.

Water

Try to drink six to eight glasses of pure water a day. Use bottled water or get a home water purifier if your tap water tastes of chlorine or other contaminants or you live in an area where the water is suspected of being contaminated. I recommend that you drink tea regularly for its antioxidant effects, especially green tea. Decaffeinated forms are available.

If you drink alcohol, red wine is probably the best choice because of the antioxidant effect of the red pigments. I do not recommend using any form of alcohol excessively or on a daily basis.

The recipe section of this book, along with the suggested menu plans, contain recommendations that are fully consistent with the optimum diet.

APPENDIX B

DIETARY RECOMMENDATIONS FOR COMMON HEALTH CONCERNS

Early in this book I quoted Hippocrates's advice to "let food be your medicine and medicine be your food" and expressed my hope that in the future doctors will be trained to prescribe dietary changes as methods both to prevent and to treat disease. Meanwhile, I would like to give you some specific dietary recommendations for common health concerns. Many of the ideas will be familiar to you from previous chapters. Remember that in the Integrative Medicine treatment plan I favor, this advice would be accompanied by recommendations about dietary supplements, exercise, stress reduction, and mind/body interactions, as well as conventional medical approaches.

These are the purely dietary changes I recommend to people who consult me about the following conditions:

ALLERGY

- Decrease protein toward 10 percent of daily caloric intake.
- Replace animal protein as much as possible with plant protein.
- Eliminate milk and milk products, substituting other calcium sources.
- Eat organically grown fruits and vegetables as much as possible as well as organic products made from wheat and soy.

ANEMIA (IRON DEFICIENCY)

- Increase consumption of healthy forms of red meat or dried beans, dried fruit, leafy greens, molasses, and cocoa.

- Take some vitamin C (100 milligrams) with meals featuring iron-rich foods.
- Do some cooking in cast-iron skillets.

ARTHRITIS

- See entries under Allergy and Inflammation.

ASTHMA

- Follow the recommendations under Allergy.
- Follow the recommendations under Inflammation.
- Experiment with eliminating (one at a time) wheat, corn, soy, and sugar for six to eight weeks to see if the condition improves.
- Eat ginger and turmeric regularly for their anti-inflammatory effects.

ATHLETE'S FOOT (AND OTHER FUNGAL INFECTIONS)

- Decrease sugar in all forms.
- Eat garlic regularly (preferably fresh, lightly cooked in dishes, or raw in salad dressings and other preparations).

AUTOIMMUNITY

- Follow the recommendations under Allergy.
- Follow the recommendations under Inflammation.

BLADDER PROBLEMS
(RECURRENT CYSTITIS AND RELATED DISORDERS)

- Avoid alcohol, coffee, decaffeinated coffee, and red and black pepper.
- Decrease sugar in all forms.

BODY ODOR

- Avoid coffee and other forms of caffeine.
- Decrease animal foods in the diet.

BRONCHITIS

- Eliminate milk and milk products, substituting other sources of calcium.
- Eat garlic regularly for its antibiotic effects.
- Eat fresh horseradish, wasabi (Japanese horseradish), and hot mustard regularly to help liquefy bronchial secretions.

BURSITIS

- Follow the recommendations under Inflammation.

CANCER PREVENTION

- Avoid polyunsaturated vegetable oils, margarine, vegetable shortening, all partially hydrogenated oils, and all foods (such as deep-fried foods) that might contain *trans*-fatty acids.
- Increase omega-3 fatty acids.
- Reduce animal foods.
- Use only hormone-free, organically produced meat, poultry, and dairy products.
- Eat plenty of fresh fruits and vegetables.
- Eat soy foods regularly.
- Use organically grown produce whenever possible.
- Eat shiitake, enokidake, maitake, and oyster mushrooms frequently.
- Drink green tea regularly.

CHOLESTEROL PROBLEMS

- Keep saturated fat intake low: no more than 5 percent of daily caloric intake.
- Increase omega-3 fatty acids, especially from fish.
- Minimize consumption of refined carbohydrates.
- Increase consumption of soluble fiber, such as oat bran.
- Eat garlic, hot red pepper (chile), and shiitake mushrooms frequently.
- Drink green tea regularly.
- Eat plenty of fresh fruits and vegetables, including leafy greens, orange and yellow fruits and vegetables, and red and purple fruits.
- Eat soy foods and other legumes regularly.

CHRONIC FATIGUE SYNDROME

- Decrease protein to 10 percent of daily caloric intake.
- Eat a variety of fresh fruits and vegetables for their protective phytochemicals.
- Eat garlic regularly for its antibiotic effects.
- Eat immune-enhancing mushrooms regularly: shiitake, oyster, enokidake, maitake.

CONSTIPATION

- Increase consumption of fiber by eating more fruits, vegetables, nuts, seeds, and whole grains.
- Drink more water.

DIABETES

- Read up on glycemic index and make an effort to implement the advice about carbohydrates in chapter 2.

DIARRHEA

- Avoid milk and milk products, raw vegetables and fruits, bran, whole-grain cereals, sugary foods, spices, caffeine, and alcohol until the problem subsides.

DIVERTICULITIS

- Increase dietary fiber in the form of wheat bran, high-fiber cereals, flax seeds, or psyllium, and drink plenty of water.
- Avoid eating raw vegetables until the acute problem subsides.
- Avoid all sources of caffeine.

EAR INFECTIONS
(RECURRENT OTITIS MEDIA IN CHILDREN)

- Eliminate milk and milk products for three months to see if the problem subsides. Calcium-fortified soy milk and soy products can be substituted.

ECZEMA

- Follow the recommendations under Allergy.
- Increase omega-3 fatty acids.

EYE PROBLEMS
(CATARACT, MACULAR DEGENERATION)

- Eat plenty of fresh fruits and vegetables for their antioxidant effects.

FIBROCYSTIC BREASTS

- Eliminate all sources of caffeine.
- Decrease dietary fat to 25 percent of daily caloric intake.
- Use only hormone-free meats, poultry, and dairy products.
- Eat soy foods regularly.

FIBROMYALGIA

- Follow the recommendations about fats under Inflammation.
- Eat ginger and turmeric regularly.

GALLBLADDER DISEASE

- Reduce dietary fat to 25 percent of daily caloric intake.
- Reduce dietary cholesterol to no more than 300 milligrams a day.
- Reduce animal foods.
- Eat soy foods regularly.
- Eat calcium-rich foods.

GOUT

- Reduce animal foods.
- Keep protein intake low, about 10 percent of daily caloric intake.
- Eliminate all caffeine sources.
- Minimize consumption of alcohol.

HEART DISEASE (CORONARY HEART DISEASE, CONGESTIVE HEART FAILURE)

- Consider a low-fat, vegetarian diet as part of a comprehensive, heart-healthy lifestyle program.
- Decrease animal foods and saturated fat.
- Follow the recommendations about fats under Cancer Prevention.
- Increase omega-3 fatty acids, especially EPA from fish and fortified eggs.
- Decrease refined carbohydrates.
- Eat plenty of fresh fruits and vegetables for their antioxidant and other protective effects.
- Eat whole grains, nuts, and seeds for their fiber and other protective factors.
- Eat soy foods regularly.
- Eat garlic regularly.
- Eat shiitake and oyster mushrooms frequently.

HYPERTENSION

- Increase fruits and vegetables.
- Avoid salted and salty foods, such as processed foods.
- Eat garlic regularly, one to two cloves a day.

HYPOGLYCEMIA

- Avoid high-glycemic-index carbohydrate foods.
- Include a low-glycemic-index carbohydrate at every meal.

IMMUNE DEFICIENCY

- Eat plenty of fresh, organically grown fruits and vegetables.
- Eat immune-enhancing mushrooms: shiitake, enokidake, maitake, and oyster.
- Follow the recommendations about fats under Cancer Prevention.

INFLAMMATION

- Eliminate polyunsaturated vegetable oils, margarine, vegetable shortening, all partially hydrogenated oils, all foods (such as deep-fried foods) that might contain *trans*-fatty acids.
- Use extra-virgin olive oil as your main fat.
- Increase intake of omega-3 fatty acids.
- Eat more fruits and vegetables.
- Eat ginger and turmeric regularly.

INFLAMMATORY BOWEL DISEASE
(ULCERATIVE COLITIS, CROHN'S DISEASE)

- Eliminate milk and milk products.
- Eliminate all caffeine sources.
- Avoid products sweetened with sorbitol or xylitol.
- During active flare-ups, avoid raw fruits and vegetables, seeds, and nuts.
- Rice gruel may be soothing and easily digested during active flare-ups.

IRRITABLE BOWEL SYNDROME

- Eliminate milk and milk products.
- Eliminate all caffeine sources.
- Increase dietary fiber by eating more whole grains, bran cereal, fruits, and vegetables.
- Avoid products sweetened with sorbitol or xylitol.

KIDNEY PROBLEMS

- Decrease protein to 10 percent or less of daily caloric intake.
- Replace animal protein in diet with vegetable protein, such as soy.

Liver Problems

- Decrease protein to 10 percent or less of daily caloric intake.
- Limit dietary fat to 25 percent of daily caloric intake.

Menstrual Problems (PMS, Dysmenorrhea)

- Follow the recommendations about fats under Inflammation.
- Use only hormone-free meats, poultry, and dairy products.
- Eat soy foods regularly.
- Eliminate all sources of caffeine.

Menopause

- Eat soy foods regularly.
- Eat calcium-rich foods.

Migraine

- Experiment with avoidance of common dietary triggers: chocolate, red wine, strong-flavored cheeses, fermented foods, sardines, anchovies, pickled herring, and cured meats.
- Eliminate all sources of caffeine.

Mood Disorders
(Mood Swings, Bipolar Disorder)

- Increase intake of omega-3 fatty acids, especially DHA from fish or fortified eggs.

Multiple Sclerosis

- Follow the recommendations under Allergy.
- Follow the recommendations under Inflammation.

Osteoarthritis

- Follow the recommendations under Inflammation.

Osteoporosis

- Decrease dietary protein.
- Replace animal protein with vegetable protein.
- Eat soy foods regularly.
- Eat broccoli and leafy greens for their content of vitamin K, which is protective of bones.

PREGNANCY

- In the last trimester, be sure to increase intake of omega-3 fatty acids, especially DHA from fish or fortified eggs.

PROSTATE PROBLEMS

- Decrease intake of animal foods and saturated fat.
- Eat soy foods regularly.
- Follow the recommendations about fats under Cancer Prevention.
- Eat plenty of fresh fruits and vegetables, including cooked tomatoes (in tomato sauce made with olive oil, for example).
- Eat whole grains, nuts, and seeds, especially raw (or freshly toasted) pumpkin seeds.
- In the case of prostatitis, avoid all caffeine sources, alcohol, black and red pepper.
- Drink green tea or use a decaffeinated green tea extract.

RHEUMATOID ARTHRITIS

- Follow the recommendations under Allergy.
- Follow the recommendations under Inflammation.

SINUS PROBLEMS

- Eliminate milk and milk products for at least two months to see how the condition responds.

STOMACH PROBLEMS

- Eliminate all caffeine sources and decaffeinated coffee.
- Reduce or eliminate alcohol.
- Eat ginger regularly.

THYROID PROBLEMS

- Eat sea vegetables to provide iodine.
- Limit intake of soy since it can interfere with thyroid function.

ULCER (PEPTIC ULCER DISEASE)

- Eat smaller, more frequent meals.
- Avoid all caffeine sources and decaffeinated coffee.
- Avoid alcohol.
- Avoid milk and milk products.

- Eat plenty of fresh fruits and vegetables.
- Experiment with hot red (chile) pepper, which promotes healing of ulcers.

URINARY PROBLEMS
- Avoid all caffeine sources.

UTERINE FIBROIDS
- Eat only hormone-free meats, poultry, and dairy products.
- Eat soy foods regularly.
- Limit dietary fat to 25 percent of daily caloric intake and follow the recommendations about fats under Cancer Prevention.
- Eat plenty of organically grown fruits and vegetables.

APPENDIX C

ANSWERS TO COMMON QUESTIONS ABOUT FOOD AND NUTRITION

How can I lose weight? I've tried everything.

Read over the information in chapter 5. Determine how many calories you are now taking in per day on average and resolve to eat less and exercise more. A good form of exercise is a forty-five-minute brisk daily walk. Eat less by decreasing the size of your portions and minimizing consumption of high-fat foods and high-glycemic-index carbohydrates. Make sure the food you do eat adheres to the nutritional guidelines in this book, satisfies your hunger, gives you pleasure.

It seems as if I gain weight just by looking at food. Why?

You may have inherited thrifty genes that give you the ability to store up calories efficiently as fat. This genetic inheritance may make you carbohydrate-sensitive, so pay special attention to the information about carbohydrates in chapter 2, section II. Keep your total carbohydrate intake to 50 percent of daily caloric intake and try to avoid high-glycemic-index carbohydrate foods, especially foods containing sugar and flour.

I've had cancer. What foods should I avoid?

Avoid foods known to be carcinogenic, such as peanuts, raw legume sprouts, common button mushrooms, cured meats, and grilled meats that are charred on the outside. Pay particular attention to the information about fats in chapter 2, section III, and stay away from polyunsaturated vegetable oils, all foods made with margarine or partially hydrogenated oils, and sources of *trans*-fatty acids. Do not eat fried foods in restaurants. Reduce your intake of animal foods and move toward a more plant-based diet. Eat plenty of fresh fruits and vegetables, preferably organic.

I have no energy. Could my diet be the problem?

Possibly. Try eating less protein and fat, fewer high-glycemic-index carbohydrates, and more fruits and vegetables. Other common causes of low energy are lack of exercise and sleep, dependence on caffeine, and depression.

I thought we were supposed to avoid dietary fat. Now I'm hearing that fat is okay and carbohydrates are bad. What are the answers?

Read the information on fat and carbohydrates in chapter 2. Your diet should contain both of these macronutrients, but it is important to know which fats are healthy and which are not and which carbohydrates are better and which are worse. The optimum diet can contain 30 percent of daily caloric intake as fat, possibly more if the fat is predominately monounsaturated and provides enough omega-3 fatty acids. It can also contain up to 60 percent of daily caloric intake as carbohydrates, preferably low-glycemic-index carbohydrates such as fruits, starchy vegetables, and foods made from whole grains.

Is it okay to eat soybeans if I had breast cancer?

The scientific evidence is not yet in on this question, so I can only give my opinion. I believe the phytoestrogens in soy (isoflavones) protect estrogen receptors from excessive stimulation by the body's own hormones and foreign estrogen-like substances. Therefore, I recommend eating soy to women at risk for breast cancer as well as those who have had it. You can eat three or four servings of soy foods a week, preferably less-processed ones made from organic soybeans.

If I change my diet, can I get off all the drugs I'm taking for my arthritis?

Possibly. The mainstream Western diet promotes inflammation. By adjusting the fats you eat and increasing intake of anti-inflammatory foods, you may be able to reduce inflammation naturally and, at least, reduce the dosages of the drugs. See the entry for Arthritis in Appendix B.

My five-year-old has asthma. Are there foods he shouldn't be eating? My doctor doesn't seem to know.

It would be worth doing some experiments with diet. The first would be to eliminate milk and all products made from milk for at least two months to see if improvement occurs. A naturopathic doctor or practitioner of traditional Chinese medicine can recommend further dietary changes.

A holistic doctor told me I'm allergic to wheat. What does that mean? I love bread and pasta.

The protein in wheat, gluten, is a not uncommon allergen. But to determine whether it is really affecting you, you would have to eliminate all wheat for a month or two, then add it back to see if you can make any correlation with symptoms. If you find that you are sensitive to wheat, you can buy gluten-free bread and pasta made from rice and corn at natural food stores.

If I'm eating pretty well, do I need to take vitamins?

I think everyone can benefit from taking supplements of the principal antioxidant vitamins and minerals (C, E, mixed carotenoids, and selenium), as well as a B complex. Many people should also supplement with calcium and vitamin D. See chapter 2, section V.

If I'm supposed to be eating more fruits and vegetables, do I have to worry about pesticides on them?

I'm afraid you do. See pages 142–3.

I don't have time to cook. How can I eat a healthy diet?

Look in natural food stores or natural food sections of supermarkets for frozen and quick-to-prepare foods that conform to the guidelines in this book—for example, instant soups, rice and bean dishes in cups, frozen entrées, and so forth. Also, find restaurants that serve healthy food (see pages 196–7). Also, try to spend more time with people who eat well. And visit the *Ask Dr. Weil* Web site for tips and group support: *www.drweil.com*.

My children like only macaroni and cheese. How can I get them to develop better eating habits?

Try to set good examples for them, because eating habits of early life often persist into adulthood. Keep trying to create tasty dishes that are also healthful, like the desserts in the recipes section of this book. If your kids won't eat broccoli, maybe they will eat stuffed baked potatoes, mixed with finely chopped broccoli, soy milk, and cheese (see page 244).

I love chocolate. Is it bad for me?

Good-quality dark chocolate is not unhealthy and makes a pleasant dessert or treat. It contains a stimulant drug that can affect some people adversely, but it has an acceptable fat content and protective phytochemicals with antioxidant activity. Dark chocolate from Belgium and France is particularly good.

The cafeteria food at my school is wretched. How can I persuade the school to improve it?

The school will probably put the blame on the food services company that has the contract to provide food for the cafeteria. Complain! And get others, including parents, to complain. If the school is publicly funded, write to your legislators. Meantime, bring your own food.

Is sugar bad for you?

Not if you are not carbohydrate-sensitive and eat it moderately. Most Americans eat way too much sugar, and it adds to the total glycemic load of their diets. Excessive consumption of sugar elevates serum triglycerides, can contribute to atherosclerosis, and can worsen insulin resistance in those who are genetically programmed for it. Anyone who eats too much sugar has a higher risk of developing dental caries.

Are microwave ovens safe?

Unless they are damaged, microwave ovens do not leak microwave radiation. But because microwaves can drive plastic molecules into food, you should only microwave food in glass or ceramic containers and never in plastic or plastic wrap. You should also be aware that microwaves can change the chemistry of food, especially proteins, possibly lowering nutritional content and possibly creating unnatural compounds that may be hazardous to health. I recommend microwave ovens for rapid heating or defrosting of food, not for cooking of more than a few minutes' duration.

Is it all right to eat eggs if heart disease runs in your family?

Yes, provided that you cook them in healthful ways—i.e., without a lot of saturated fat. I strongly recommend using the new omega-3 fortified eggs from free-range chickens. The essential fatty acids in the yolks are very protective of the heart and arteries.

Is it dangerous to cook in aluminum pots?

Maybe, depending on what you are cooking. If you cook acidic foods in them, such as tomatoes, aluminum can get into the foods and therefore into your body, where it probably does no good. Pots with aluminum exteriors for better heat conduction and stainless steel interiors are fine. But I would stay away from pots with aluminum cooking surfaces. I see no problem in broiling fish or other foods on aluminum foil, covering baking dishes with this material, or wrapping food in it for storage.

I read that dairy products could be causing my sinus problems. Isn't milk supposed to be the perfect food?

See pages 113–5 for my thoughts about problems with milk as a food. Anyone with sinus problems should try eliminating milk and all products made from milk from the diet for at least two months to see what happens. Most people who try this experiment experience significant improvement.

Are artificial sweeteners safe?

In a word, no. Nor do they help people lose weight.

Is it okay to drink water with your meals?

Yes. Water does not dilute digestive juices or otherwise interfere with digestion.

What's the best way to eat if I want to live to be a hundred?

Follow all the dietary advice in this book. In particular, eat moderately rather than excessively; minimize consumption of processed foods; and eat plenty of fresh fruits and vegetables.

APPENDIX D

THE POSSIBILITY OF SURVIVING
WITHOUT EATING

Shortly after I finished my medical training, I read a delightful book that awakened in me an interest in yoga and Indian religious philosophies: *Autobiography of a Yogi* by Paramahansa Yogananda (1893–1952). It is filled with wondrous tales from an exotic land, none more amazing than that of Giri Bala, "a woman yogi who never eats." There is a photograph of her, a little grandmother wrapped in a shawl, captioned, "She employs a certain yogic technique to recharge her body with cosmic energy from the ether, sun, and air." Yogananda made a visit to Bala's home in northern Bengal in 1936 and recorded her story.

As a child Bala was given to gluttony. She prayed for salvation and met a guru who initiated her into an esoteric practice "that frees the body from dependence on the gross food of mortals." She told Yogananda, "The technique includes the use of a certain *mantra* and a breathing exercise more difficult than the average person could perform. No medicine or magic is involved. . . ."

"Mother," asked Yogananda, "what is the use of your having been singled out to live by the Eternal Light and not by food?"

"To prove that man is Spirit. To demonstrate that by divine advancement he can gradually learn to live by the Eternal Light and not by food."

In my own research I have not encountered this technique or any direct evidence of its existence. When I was living in South America in the early 1970s, I ran into a number of seekers on the trail of the "Breatharians," a supposed sect of noneaters, who had their headquarters in a hidden monastery near the shore of Lake Titicaca, where they lived on air and cosmic energy, having passed through preliminary stages of vegetarianism and fruitarianism. No one I met had found this place, but some years later I was amused to learn of the exposure of a self-proclaimed Breatharian guru in California, captured on videotape stuffing himself with candy between lectures.

But there is a spectacular, large-scale revival of claims for living without food by the mostly Chinese followers of a modern *qigong* master, Yan Xin. The fact that his disciples are mostly doctors, researchers, engineers, and other well-educated people, many of them working in the West, makes their stories of having not eaten in months or years somewhat more compelling and accessible. *Qigong* is an ancient Chinese practice intended to increase the body's stores of *qi* (chi), universal life energy, to promote its internal circulation in order to improve health and vitality, and to direct it outward as a healing method or a force to affect physical objects. It makes use of exercises, breathing techniques, and mental and spiritual disciplines. Yan Xin is one of the more dramatic and puzzling adepts to come to the West, a leader in the recent revival of interest in *qigong* that followed on the decline of hard-line communism in China. He frequently demonstrates the ability to affect physical systems by "emitting" *qi*, which he says takes tremendous energy. Yan Xin encourages scientific investigation of his powers and methods, and his adherents have published a great many experimental studies in a variety of academic journals (summaries of them may be found on the Web page of the International Yan Xin Qigong Association at *http://www.qigong.net*).

One of Yan Xin's interests is production of an altered physiological state called *bigu*, meaning "abstention from food," by means of his *qigong* practice. At large conventions in New York in 1997 and 1998, some of his followers, all Chinese and almost all with "M.D." or "Ph.D." after their names, described their attainment of this state in talks with titles like "My Understanding about Bigu Phenomenon," "My Bigu Experience," and "My Bigu Journey." They said they could enter and leave the state, and when in it, not eat at all or eat and drink very little for extended periods.

One spokeswoman, Jun Wang, Ph.D., a thirty-four-year-old electrical engineer who works as a software developer for a computer company in New Jersey, has been in the abstaining-from-food state for eight years. She told me:

I went to one of Yan Xin's lectures when I was a graduate student at the University of Connecticut. Of course, I had heard about *qigong* growing up in China. Yan Xin talked a lot about *qigong* theory and the experiments being done to test it, and he also emitted *qi* during his lecture. I had no reaction, but I saw a lot of reactions in others, including spontaneous healing of health problems. It was amazing. He mentioned *bigu,* and I have since learned the technique. I have been told not to reveal it, but I can say it involves adjusting the mind and thoughts, especially cultivating the virtue principle, and is a twenty-four-hour-a-day practice.

I joined the University of Connecticut chapter of the Yan Xin Qigong Society and began to practice. The early stages of the work are relatively simple, the advanced stages relatively difficult. I stopped eating regular food; I didn't feel hungry. Instead I drank water, tea, or juice, and I've continued that way ever since. I feel perfect, have much energy, and no health problems.

Shortly after starting the *bigu* state I went to a conference where my colleagues wanted to go out to dinner every night. I sat with them at meals for a whole week but just took water.

I believe about a thousand people have had similar experiences. Some go in and out of the state. I believe I still get energy from some source. The practice has helped me receive and preserve energy, and, I think, develop a new source of energy in my body.

Please bear in mind that I am simply reporting secondhand information here, that I have no direct experience of *bigu,* and cannot vouch for the veracity of any of this material. I would very much like to know if the studies done by Yan Xin's followers can be replicated by disinterested Western scientists and whether the *bigu* state is real. If so, it is, at least, an anomaly not explainable by prevailing scientific and medical paradigms.

APPENDIX E

SOURCES OF INFORMATION, MATERIALS, AND SUPPLIES

BOOKS

Alford, Jeffrey, and Naomi Duguid. *Seductions of Rice: A Cookbook.* New York: Artisan, 1998.

Aronne, Lou, M.D. *Weigh Less, Live Longer: Dr. Lou Aronne's "Getting Healthy" Plan for Permanent Weight Control.* Chichester: John Wiley & Sons, 1997.

Brand-Miller, Jennie, Thomas M. S. Wolever, Stephen Colagiuri, and Kaye Foster-Powell. *The Glucose Revolution: The Authoritative Guide to the Glycemic Index.* New York: Marlowe & Co., 1999.

Carper, Jean. *Food Your Miracle Medicine.* London: Simon & Schuster, 2000.

Emmons, Didi. *Vegetarian Planet: 350 Big-Flavor Recipes for Out-of-This-World Food Every Day.* Boston: Harvard Common Press, 1997.

Fletcher, Anne M., and Graham Kerr. *Eating Thin for Life: Food Secrets and Recipes from People Who Have Lost Weight and Kept It Off.* New York: Chapters, 1998.

Gelenberg, Patricia, and Helen Newton Hartung. *The Whole Soy Cookbook: 175 Delicious, Nutritious, Easy-to-Prepare Recipes Featuring Tofu, Tempeh, and Various Forms of Nature's Healthiest Bean.* New York: Random House, 1998.

Goldbeck, Nikki, and David Goldbeck. *The Healthiest Diet in the World: A Cookbook and Mentor.* New York: Dutton, 1998.

The Green Food Shopper: An Activist's Guide to Changing the Food System. New York: Mothers & Others for a Livable Planet, 1997.

Jacobi, Dana. *The Natural Kitchen: Soy!: 75 Delicious Ways to Enjoy Nature's Miracle Food.* Rocklin, California: Prima, 1996.

Jenkins, Nancy Harmon, and Antonia Trichopoulou. *The Mediterranean Diet Cookbook: A Delicious Alternative for Lifelong Health.* New York: Bantam Doubleday Dell, 1994.

Kesten, Deborah. *Feeding the Body, Nourishing the Soul.* Berkeley, California: Conari Press, 1997.

McCully, Kilmer, M.D. *The Homocysteine Revolution: Medicine for the New Millennium.* New Canaan, Connecticut: Keats Publishing, 1997.

Mitscher, Lester A., and Victoria Dolby. *The Green Tea Book.* Garden City Park, New York: Avery, 1998.

The Moosewood Collective. *Moosewood Restaurant Low-Fat Favorites: Flavorful Recipes for Healthful Meals.* New York: Clarkson Potter, 1996.

Pitchford, Paul. *Healing with Whole Foods: Oriental Traditions and Modern Nutrition.* Berkeley, California: North Atlantic Books, 1993.

Sass, Lorna L. *Lorna Sass' Short-Cut Vegetarian: Great Taste in No Time.* New York: Quill/Morrow 1997.

Schulman, Martha Rose. *Mediterranean Light: Delicious Recipes from the World's Healthiest Cuisine.* New York: Bantam, 1989.

Simonds, Nina. *A Spoonful of Ginger: Irresistible, Health-Giving Recipes from Asian Kitchens.* Bath: Absolute Press, 2000.

Simopoulos, Artemis P., M.D., and Jo Robinson. *The Omega Diet: The Lifelong Nutritional Program Based on the Diet of the Island of Crete.* New York: HarperCollins, 1999.

Wood, Rebecca, et al. *The New Whole Foods Encyclopedia: A Comprehensive Resource for Healthy Living.* New York: Penguin USA, 1999.

Zipern, Elizabeth, and Dar Williams. *The Tofu Tollbooth.* Woodstock, New York: Ceres Press, 1998.

MAGAZINES

Cooking Light   *Natural Health*   *Vegetarian Times*

WEB SITES

Ask Dr. Weil:
www.drweil.com

Campaign for Food Safety:
www.purefood.org

International Slow Food Movement:
www.slowfood.com

Mothers and Others for a Livable Planet:
www.mothers.org/mothers

Mothers for Natural Law:
www.safe-food.org

U.S.D.A. Food and Nutrition Information Center:
www.nal.usda.gov/fnic

The Vegetarian Resource Group:
www.vrg.org

NEWSLETTERS

Dr. Andrew Weil's Self-Healing
(800) 523-3296

Environmental Nutrition
(800) 829-5384

Nutrition Action Healthletter
(202) 332-9110

Tufts University Health & Nutrition Letter (800) 274-7581

ORGANIZATIONS

Center for Science in the Public
  Interest
1875 Connecticut Avenue NW—
  Suite 300
Washington, D.C. 20009
(202) 332-9110
www.cspinet.org/home.html
Publishes *Nutrition Action Newsletter*

Community Alliance with Family
  Farmers
P.O. Box 363
Davis, California 95617
(916) 756-8518
www.caff.org
Promotes community agriculture and
  publishes the *National Organic
  Directory*

Environmental Working Group
1718 Connecticut Avenue NW—
  Suite 600
Washington, D.C. 20009
(202) 667-6982
Provides information about dangers
  of agrichemicals

Mothers and Others for a Livable
  Planet
40 West 20th Street
New York, New York 10011-4211
(888) 326-4636
www.mothers.org/mothers
Promotes sustainable and organic
  agriculture

MAIL-ORDER SOURCES

Corti Brothers
P.O. Box 191358
Sacramento, California 95819
(916) 736-3800
Organic olive oils

Frieda's
4465 Corporate Center Drive
Los Alamitos, California 90720
(800) 241-1771
www.friedas.com
Specialty fruits and vegetables

Fungi Perfecti
P.O. Box 7634
Olympia, Washington 98507
(800) 780-9126
www.fungi.com
Gourmet and medicinal mushrooms

Gold Mine Natural Food Company
7805 Arjons Drive
San Diego, California 92126-4368
(800) 475-3663
www.goldminesnatural.com
Organic grains, nuts, beans, sea
  vegetables

Heintzman Farms
RR 2, Box 265
Onaka, South Dakota 57466
(800) 333-5813
Flax seeds and grinders

The Mail Order Catalog for Healthy
  Eating
P.O. Box 180
Summertown, Tennessee 38483
(800) 835-2867
www.healthy-eating.com
Vegetarian cookbooks and products

Maine Coast Sea Vegetables
RR 1, Box 78
Franklin, Maine 04634
(207) 565-2907
www.seaveg.com
Sea vegetables

The Ohio Hempery, Inc.
P.O. Box 18
Guysville, Ohio 45735
(800) 289-4367
www.hempery.com/main.html
Hemp seeds and oil
Oriental Pantry

423 Great Road
Acton, Massachusetts 01720
(800) 828-0368
Asian cooking supplies

Zingerman's
422 Detroit Street
Ann Arbor, Michigan 48104-3400
(888) 636-8162
Organic olive oils, cheeses

UNITED KINGDOM

INFORMATION ON WATER

Try your Environmental Health
Office — please contact your local
council (or Scottish Environmental
Health Office or the Water Service of
the Department of the Environment
for Northern Ireland).

You can also contact the local
Customer Services Committee of
OFWAT (see telephone directory).
Ask for their Customer Code of Practice for their complaints procedure.

INFORMATION ON ORGANIC PRODUCE

Soil Association
Bristol House
40–56 Victoria Street
Bristol BS1 6BY
0117 929 0661

SUPPLIERS

Nature's Best Health Products
Century Place
Tunbridge Wells
Kent TN2 3BE
Orders: 01892 552117
One of the largest mail-order suppliers of nutritional supplements with
over 160 products in their range.
They have a nutritional advice hotline
on 01892 552118.

Neal's Yard
29 John Dalton Street
Manchester M2 6DS
0161 831 7875
Supplies a wide range of food supplements, herbs, tonics, essential oils.
Mail-order catalogue available.

OTHER USEFUL
ADDRESSES

Consumers' Association (*Which?*
magazine)
2 Marylebone Road
London NW1
020 7830 6000

Friends of the Earth
26–28 Underwood Street
London N1 7JQ
020 7490 1555

NOTES

1. THE PRINCIPLES OF EATING WELL

5 American Council on Science and Health: *Medical Tribune*, 21 January 1999, p. 20.

6 Super blue-green algae: "Did You Know? Some Interesting Facts About Super Blue Green Algae," Cell Tech Company, Klamath Falls, Oregon, 1998.

11 ... food and eating modify neurochemistry: C. Prasad, "Food, Mood, and Health: A Neurobiologic Outlook," *Brazilian Journal of Medical and Biological Research* 31 (12), 1517–27, 1998.

12 Here is a snapshot of one prodigious eater: Brendan Gill, *Here at the New Yorker* (New York: Da Capo Press, 1997), pp. 322–23.

13 Consider this recipe: Nomi Shannon, *The Raw Gourmet: Simple Recipes for Living Well* (Vancouver: Alive Books, 1999), p. 132.

14 Ronald Koetzsch: Ronald Koetzsch, "Camaraderie Is the Best Diet," *Natural Health*: Jan./Feb. 1994, pp. 151–52. Used by permission.

18 Wade Davis: quoted in "Explorers of the Millennium," *National Geographic Adventure*: Spring 1999 (premiere issue), p. 94.

18 ... combinations of ingredients ... that provide instantly recognizable textures, flavors, and aromas: Elizabeth Rozin, "The Structure of Cuisine," in L. M. Baker (ed.), *The Psychobiology of Human Food Selection* (Westport, Connecticut: AVI Publishing, 1982). *See also,* Elizabeth Rozin, *Ethnic Cuisine: The Flavor-Principle Cookbook* (Brattleboro, Vermont: The Stephen Greene Press, 1983).

18 (footnote) Authorities differ about the existence of human societies that practice cannibalism: W. Arens, *The Man-Eating Myth: Anthropology and Anthropophagy* (New York: Oxford University Press, 1979); G. Kolata, "Anthropologists Suggest Cannibalism Is a Myth," *Science* 232, 1497–1500, 1986; P. Villa et al., "Cannibalism in the Neolithic," *Science* 233, 431–38, 1986.

21 . . . deaths from heart attacks dropped precipitously: H. Malmros, "Diet, Lipids, and Atherosclerosis," *Acta Medica Scandinavica* 207 (3), 145–49, 1980.

21 Japanese women on traditional diets: S. Tominaga and T. Kuroishi, "Epidemiology of Breast Cancer in Japan," *Cancer Letters* 90 (1), 75–79, 1995.

21 Japanese men on traditional diets: T. Hirayama, "Epidemiology of Prostate Cancer with Special Reference to the Role of Diet," *National Cancer Institute Monographs* 53, 149–55, 1979.

22 Studies of Seventh Day Adventists: R. L. Phillips et al., "Coronary Heart Disease Mortality Among Seventh Day Adventists with Differing Dietary Habits: A Preliminary Report," *American Journal of Clinical Nutrition* 31 (10 supplement), S191–98, 1978; G. E. Fraser et al., "Ischemic Heart Disease Risk Factors in Middle-Aged Seventh-Day Adventist Men and Their Neighbors," *American Journal of Epidemiology* 126 (4), 638–46, 1987.

22 . . . the University of Arizona's Program in Integrative Medicine: For information, visit the Program's Web site at *http://integrativemedicine. arizona.edu*

23 Nina Simonds . . . described a visit: Nina Simonds, *A Spoonful of Ginger: Irresistible, Health-Giving Recipes from Asian Kitchens* (New York: Alfred A. Knopf, 1999), pp. 23–25.

2. THE BASICS OF HUMAN NUTRITION

31 The Atkins diet: *See* Robert C. Atkins, M.D., *Dr. Atkins' Diet Revolution* (New York: Bantam, 1973).

32 . . . the Montignac diet: *See* Michel Montignac, *Dine Out and Lose Weight* (Los Angeles: Montignac USA, Inc., 1995).

32 Dean Ornish: *See* Dean Ornish, M.D., *Eat More, Weigh Less* (New York: Harper Perennial Library, 1994). *See also*, "Fat Fight" (a debate between Dr. Ornish and Dr. Atkins), *Natural Health*, June 1999, p. 98.

32 "That's ridiculous," Atkins retorts: Robert C. Atkins, M.D., personal communication, May 6, 1999.

32 The Zone: *See* Barry Sears, Ph.D., *Enter the Zone* (New York: Harper-Collins, 1995).

35 "You might say . . .": "Fat Fight," *Natural Health*, June 1999, p. 101.

36 But the biochemistry text I read: Thomas M. Devlin, ed., *Textbook of Biochemistry with Clinical Correlations, 4th Ed.* (New York: Wiley & Sons, 1997), p. 1108.

44 Here is how I described them in my book *Spontaneous Healing*: Andrew Weil, M.D., *Spontaneous Healing: How to Discover and Enhance Your Body's Natural Ability to Maintain and Heal Itself* (New York: Alfred A. Knopf, 1995), p. 73.

50 . . . human nutrition in truly ancient times: S. Boyd Eaton, M.D., and Stan-

ley B. Eaton III, "Evolution, Diet, and Health," unpublished manuscript, Departments of Anthropology and Radiology, Emory University, 1999.

50 We are told that the advent of agriculture: S. Boyd Eaton, M.D., and Stanley B. Eaton III, "Evolution, Diet, and Health." *See also,* W. J. Lutz, "The Colonization of Europe and Our Western Diseases," *Medical Hypotheses* 45 (2), 115–20, 1995.

52 To measure glycemic index: Jennie Brand-Miller, Thomas M. S. Wolever, Stephen Colagiuri, and Kaye Foster-Powell, *The Glucose Revolution: The Authoritative Guide to the Glycemic Index* (New York: Marlowe & Company, 1999), pp. 26–27.

58 . . . the amounts [of carrots] that people do eat contribute only moderately to the rise in blood sugar: Brand-Miller et al., *Glucose Revolution,* p. 54.

58 *Sugar Busters:* H. Leighton Steward, *Sugar Busters* (New York: Ballantine, 1998).

58 *Sugar Blues:* William Duffy, *Sugar Blues* (New York: Warner Books, 1993).

60 "Food preparation was a simple process": Brand-Miller et al., *Glucose Revolution,* p. 3.

60 . . . the sources of carbohydrate in our diets today: Brand-Miller et al., *Glucose Revolution,* p. 13.

62 Corn syrup is a more recent invention: Carl Reeder, Archer Daniels Midland Corporation, personal communication, July 1999.

63 Polynesians: *See* Terry Shintani, *Dr. Shintani's Hawaii Diet* (New York: Pocket Books, 1999).

63 Pimas and O'odham (Papagos): Gary Paul Nabhan, *Cultures of Habitat* (Washington, D.C.: Counterpoint, 1997), pp. 199–206. *See also,* B. A. Swinburn et al., "Deterioration in Carbohydrate Metabolism and Lipoprotein Changes Induced by a Modern, High-Fat Diet in Pima Indians and Caucasians," *Journal of Clinical Endocrinology and Metabolism* 73 (1), 156–65, 1991; J. C. Brand et al., "Plasma Glucose and Insulin Response to Traditional Pima Indian Meals," *American Journal of Clinical Nutrition* 51 (3), 416–20, 1990.

64 . . . this disease [type II diabetes] has begun to appear in children: A. L. Rosenbloom et al., "Emerging Epidemic of Type 2 Diabetes in Youth," *Diabetes Care* 22 (2), 345–54, 1999; N. S. Glaser, "Non-insulin Dependent Diabetes Mellitus in Childhood and Adolescence," *Pediatric Clinics of North America* 44 (2), 307–37, 1997.

64 Similar experiments with native Hawaiians: Shintani, *Hawaii Diet.*

65 . . . syndrome X (insulin resistance syndrome): Gerald M. Reaven, M.D., "Pathophysiology of Insulin Resistance in Human Disease," *Physiological Reviews* 75 (3), 473–87, 1995.

65 How prevalent is carbohydrate sensitivity?: Gerald M. Reaven, M.D., personal communication, July 1999.

66 ... very high carbohydrate diets actually increase the effectiveness of insulin slightly: Gerald M. Reaven, M.D., personal communication, July 1999.

68 *Calories Don't Count:* Herman Taller, M.D., *Calories Don't Count* (New York: Simon & Schuster, 1961).

77 ... so-called Methusaleh genes: K. Berg, "Lp(a) Lipoprotein: An Overview," *Chemistry and Physics of Lipids* 9 (16), 67–68, 1994.

77 ... inclusion [of egg yolks] in the diet makes an insignificant contribution to serum cholesterol: F. B. Hu et al., "A Prospective Study of Egg Consumption and Risk of Cardiovascular Disease in Men and Women," *Journal of the American Medical Association* 281 (15), 1387–94, 1999.

78 ... or even by a bacterial infection: J. T. Grayston, "Does Chlamydia Pneumoniae Cause Atherosclerosis?" *Archives of Surgery* 134 (9), 930–34, 1999.

79 Since the late 1960s the epidemic of heart attacks has waned: National Heart, Lung, and Blood Institute, *Morbidity and Mortality: 1998 Chartbook on Cardiovascular, Lung, and Blood Diseases* (Rockville, Maryland: National Institutes of Health, 1998).

79 One possibility ... : "Decline in Deaths from Heart Disease and Stroke—United States, 1900–1999," *Morbidity and Mortality Weekly Report,* 48 (30), 649–56, 1999.

79 ... as peoples of other countries begin to eat the way we do, their rates of coronary heart disease go up: D. L. McGee et al., "Ten Year Incidence of Coronary Heart Disease in the Honolulu Heart Program: Relationship to Nutrient Intake," *American Journal of Epidemiology* 119 (5), 667–76, 1984.

80 Scotland ... has staggering rates of cardiovascular disease: R. A. Riemersma, "Dietary Fatty Acids and Antioxidant Vitamins and the Risk of Coronary Heart Disease: The Scottish Experience," *Acta Cardiologica* 44 (6), 482–83, 1989.

80 Cretans eat 40 percent of their calories as fat: Ancel Keys, *Seven Countries: A Multivariate Analysis of Death and Coronary Heart Disease* (Cambridge, Massachusetts: Harvard University Press, 1980).

83 Unless salmon farmers ... : J. Nettleton, "Comparing Nutrients in Wild and Farmed Fish, *Aquaculture Magazine,* Jan./Feb. 1999. *See also,* E. Bergstrom, "Effects of Natural and Artificial Diets on Seasonal Changes in Fatty Acid Composition and Total Body Lipid Content of Wild and Hatchery-Reared Atlantic Salmon," *Aquaculture* 82, 205–17, 1989.

83 Women ... who regularly ate mayonnaise: F. B. Hu et al., "Dietary Intake of Alpha-Linolenic Acid and Risk of Fatal Ischemic Heart Disease Among Women," *American Journal of Clinical Nutrition* 69 (5), 890–97, 1999.

86 For one key function: R. Zurier et al., "Gamma-Linolenic Acid Treatment of Rheumatoid Arthritis," *Arthritis and Rheumatism* 39 (11), 1808–17, 1996.

86 . . . daily, low-dose aspirin turns out to reduce risks: G. Morgan, "Beneficial Effects of NSAIDS in the Gastro-Intestinal Tract," *European Journal of Gastroenterology and Hepatology* 11 (4), 393–400, 1999.

87 . . . dietary intake of EFAs can affect [the balance of prostaglandins]: See Artemis Simopoulos, M.D., and Jo Robinson: *The Omega Plan* (New York: HarperCollins, 1998), p. 114. *See also,* Udo Erasmus, *Fats and Oils: The Complete Guide to Fats and Oils in Health and Nutrition* (Burnaby, British Columbia: Alive Books, 1991), pp. 255–59.

88 In April 1999 . . . : Artemis Simopoulos, M.D., Alexander Leaf, M.D., and Normal Salem, Jr., Ph.D., *Workshop on the Essentiality and Recommended Dietary Intakes for Omega-6 and Omega-3 Fatty Acids* (Rockville, Maryland: National Institutes of Health, 1999).

88 An earlier NIH meeting . . . on omega-3 fatty acids . . . and . . . mental health: Artemis Simopoulos, M.D., et al., *Workshop on Essential Fatty Acids and Psychiatric Disorders* (Bethesda, Maryland: National Institutes of Health, 1998).

89 Oxidized oils promote arterial damage: M. J. A. Williams et al., "Impaired Endothelial Function Following a Meal Rich in Used Cooking Fat," *Journal of the American College of Cardiology* 33 (4), 1050, 1999.

90 A recent research paper: ibid.

92 Margarine is made . . . : A. Ascherio et al., "Trans-Fatty Acid Intake and Risk of Myocardial Infarction," *Circulation* 89 (1), 94–101, 1994.

98 . . . the fat of marine mammals now contains high levels of toxins: M. Watanabe et al., "Contamination Levels and Specific Accumulation of Persistent Organochlorines in Caspian Seal (Phoca caspica) from the Caspian Sea, Russia," *Archives of Environmental Contamination & Toxicology* 37 (3), 396–407, 1999.

99 One outstanding danger . . . : D. M. Dreon and R. M. Krauss, "A Very-Low-Fat Diet Is Not Associated with Improved Lipoprotein Profiles in Men with a Predominance of Large Low-Density Lipoproteins," *American Journal of Clinical Nutrition* 69 (3), 411, 1999.

102 . . . cocoa butter does not raise cholesterol: Penny M. Kris-Etherton et al., "Effects of a Milk Chocolate Bar a Day Substituted for a High-Carbohydrate Snack in Young Men on an NCEP/AHA Step One Diet," *American Journal of Clinical Nutrition* 60 (6 supplement), 1037s-42s, 1994. Also, Penny M. Kris-Etherton and Vikkie A. Mustad, "Chocolate Feeding Studies: A Novel Approach for Evaluating the Plasma Lipid Effects of Stearic Acid," *American Journal of Clinical Nutrition* 60 (6 supplement), 1029s-36s, 1994.

103 *Diet for a Small Planet:* Frances Moore Lappé, *Diet for a Small Planet* (New York: Ballantine Books, 1992).

104 . . . studies consistently show [vegetarians] to be healthier and longer-lived than meat eaters: Walter C. Willett, "Convergence of Philosophy and Science: The Third International Congress on Vegetarian Nutrition,"

American Journal of Clinical Nutrition 70 (3 supplement), 434s–38s, 1999.

106 ... high-protein diets promote calcium loss: M. B. Zemel, "Calcium Utilization: Effect of Varying Level and Source of Dietary Protein," *American Journal of Clinical Nutrition* 48 (3 supplement), 880s–83s, 1988.

107 Research also suggests ... : H. M. Dosch, "The Possible Link Between Insulin Dependent (Juvenile) Diabetes Mellitus and Dietary Cow Milk," *Clinical Biochemistry* 26 (4), 307–8, 1993; S. M. Virtanen et al., "Infant Feeding in Finnish Children Less Than Seven Years Age with Newly Diagnosed IDDM," *Diabetes Care* 14 (5), 415–17, 1991.

109 mad cow disease: Richard Rhodes, *Deadly Feasts: The Prion Controversy and the Public's Health* (New York: Touchstone, 1998).

112 *Animal Liberation:* Peter Singer, *Animal Liberation* (New York: New York Review of Books, 1990).

113 ... cows and cars do almost equal damage: Michael Brower and Union of Concerned Scientists, *The Consumer's Guide to Effective Environmental Choices* (New York: Three Rivers Press, 1999).

114 ... BGH can increase rates of mastitis: Paul Kingsnorth, "Bovine Growth Hormones," *The Ecologist* 28 (5), Sep./Oct. 1998.

115 ... populations eating fish have better health and longevity than those that don't: G. Mimura et al., "Nutritional Factors for Longevity in Okinawa—Present and Future," *Nutrition and Health* 8 (2–3), 159–63, 1992. *See also,* M. Nube et al., "Scoring of Prudent Dietary Habits and Its Relation to 25-Year Survival," *Journal of the American Dietetic Association* 87 (2), 171–75, 1987.

122 ... many of these [mushrooms] offer important health benefits: R. Chang, "Functional Properties of Edible Mushrooms," *Nutrition Reviews* 54 (11, part 2), S91–93, 1996.

125 ... too much vitamin C: Anitra C. Carr and Balz Frei, "Toward a New Recommended Dietary Allowance for Vitamin C Based on Antioxidant and Health Effects in Humans," *American Journal of Clinical Nutrition* 69 (6), 1086–1107, 1999.

127 [Folic acid] is important ... in regulating levels of homocysteine: J. W. Eikelboom et al., "Homocyst(e)ine and Cardiovascular Disease: A Critical Review of the Epidemiologic Evidence," *Annals of Internal Medicine* 131 (5), 363–75, 1999. *See also,* Kilmer S. McCully, *The Homocysteine Revolution* (New Canaan, Connecticut: Keats Publishing, 1997).

129 ... vitamin E ... is now recognized: R. Brigelius-Flohe and M. G. Traber, "Vitamin E: Function and Metabolism," *Federation of American Societies for Experimental Biology (FASEB) Journal* 13 (10), 1145–55, 1999.

130 ... gamma-tocopherol is more powerful than alpha-tocopherol in preventing cancer: S. Christen et al., "Gamma-tocopherol Traps Mutagenic Electrophiles Such as NO(X) and Complements Alpha-tocopherol: Physi-

ological Implications," *Proceedings of the National Academy of Sciences* 94 (7), 3217–22, 1997.

134 Significant fractions of the population are salt-sensitive: J. P. Mtabaji et al., "Ethnic Differences in Salt Sensitivity: Genetic or Environmental Factors?" *Clinical & Experimental Pharmacology & Physiology* Supplement 20, 65–67, 1992.

135 . . . low soil selenium . . . higher cancer rates: J. C. Fleet, "Dietary Selenium Repletion May Reduce Cancer Incidence in People at High Risk Who Live in Areas with Low Soil Selenium," *Nutrition Reviews* 55 (7), 277–79, 1997.

136 . . . insoluble fibers protect the health of the intestinal tract: W. G. Bennett and J. J. Cerda, "Benefits of Dietary Fiber. Myth or Medicine?" *Postgraduate Medicine* 99 (2), 153–56, 166–68, 171–72 *passim*, 1996.

138 . . . EGCG . . . in green tea: C. S. Yang and Z. Y. Wang, "Tea and Cancer," *Journal of the National Cancer Institute* 85, 1038–49, 1993; S. K. Kattyar et al., "Polyphenolic Antioxidant (-)-Epigallocatechin-3-gallate from Green Tea Reduces UVB-induced Inflammatory Responses and Infiltration of Leukocytes in Human Skin," *Photochemistry & Photobiology* 69 (2), 148–53, 1999; F. M. Clydesdale, "Tea and Health," *Critical Reviews in Food Science and Nutrition* 36, 691–785, 1997; J. K. Lin et al., "Cancer Chemoprevention by Tea Polyphenols Through Mitotic Signal Transduction Blockade," *Biochemical Pharmacology* 58 (6), 911–15, 1999.

138 . . . red and purple pigments: X. Ye et al., "The Cytotoxic Effects of a Novel IH636 Grape Seed Proanthocyanidin Extract on Cultured Human Cancer Cells," *Molecular and Cellular Biochemistry* 196, 99–108, 1999.

139 The carotenoids: M. S. Micozzi et al., "Carotenoid Analysis of Selected Raw and Cooked Foods Associated with a Lower Risk for Cancer," *Journal of the National Cancer Institute* 82 (8), 715, 1990; T. A. Smith, "Carotenoids and Cancer: Prevention and Potential Therapy," *British Journal of Biomedical Science* 55 (4), 268–75, 1998.

139 Supplemental beta carotene might promote cancer: Olli P. Heinonen and Demetrius Albanes, "The Effect of Vitamin E and Beta-Carotene on the Incidence of Lung Cancer and Other Cancers in Male Smokers," *New England Journal of Medicine* 330 (15), 1029–35, 1994.

139 Lycopene may reduce risks of prostate cancer: E. Giovannucci, "Tomatoes, Lycopene, and Prostate Cancer," *Proceedings of the Society for Experimental Biology and Medicine* 218, 129–39, 1998; E. Giovannucci, "Tomatoes, Tomato-Based Products, Lycopene, and Cancer: Review of the Epidemiologic Literature," *Journal of the National Cancer Institute* 91, 317–31, 1999.

140 Soy isoflavones . . . : M. J. Messina, "Soy Intake and Cancer Risk: A Review of the In Vitro and In Vivo Data," *Nutrition and Cancer* 21 (2),

113–28, 1994; M. A. Moyad, "Soy, Disease Prevention, and Prostate Cancer," *Seminars in Urologic Oncology* 17 (2), 97–102, 1999.

141 Nonetheless, polysaccharides . . . : A. T. Borchers et al., "Mushrooms, Tumors, and Immunity," *Proceedings of the Society for Experimental Biology & Medicine* 221 (4), 281–93, 1999.

142 . . . wash produce before using it: H. J. Schattenberg 3rd et al., "Effects of Household Preparation on Levels of Pesticide Residues in Produce," *Journal of AOAC International* 79 (6), 1447–53, 1996.

4. THE BEST DIET IN THE WORLD

156 . . . blackened animal flesh is carcinogenic: M. G. Knize et al., "Mutagenic Activity and Heterocyclic Amine Content of the Human Diet," *Princess Takamatsu Symposia* 23, 30–38, 1995.

158 . . . percentage of healthy [Japanese] people: Joseph Coleman, "Survey: Fewer Japanese Are Healthy," *Associated Press,* August 25, 1999.

161 A recent small study of adult-onset diabetics: A. S. Nicholson et al., "Toward Improved Management of NIDDM: A Randomized Controlled, Pilot Intervention Using a Low-Fat Vegetarian Diet," *Preventive Medicine* 29 (2), 87–91, 1999.

162 Ancel Keys: Ancel B. Keys, *Eat Well, Stay Well the Mediterranean Way* (Garden City, New York: Doubleday, 1975).

5. A MATTER OF WEIGHT

173 . . . airlines have made coach seats a bit roomier: Laurence Zuckerman, "Ideas & Trends; Cramped? You're a Bit Flighty," *The New York Times* (Week in Review), 5 September 1999.

173 A survey conducted . . . : A. H. Mokdad et al., "The Spread of the Obesity Epidemic in the United States, 1991–1998," *Journal of the American Medical Association* 282 (16), 1519–22, 1999.

174 . . . the French Paradox: Malcolm Law and Nicholas Wald, "Why Heart Disease Mortality Is Low in France: The Time-Lag Explanation," *British Medical Journal* 318, 1471–80, 1999.

176 The pharmaceutical industry: P. J. Carek and L. M. Dickerson, "Current Concepts in the Pharmacological Management of Obesity," *Drugs* 57 (6), 883–904, 1999.

176 . . . leptin: C. S. Mantzoros, "The Role of Leptin in Human Obesity and Disease: A Review of Current Evidence," *Annals of Internal Medicine* 130 (8), 671–80, 1999.

177 Green chile macaroni and cheese: *The Arizona Daily Star,* 13 October 1999, Section E, p. 2.

178 . . . an appetite control center in the hypothalamus: A. W. Thorburn and J. Proietto, "Neuropeptides, the Hypothalamus, and Obesity: Insights into the Central Control of Body Weight," *Pathology* 30 (3), 229–36, 1998;

R. E. Keesey and M. D. Hirvonen, "Body Weight Set-Points: Determination and Adjustment," *Journal of Nutrition* 127 (9), 1875s-83s, 1997.

179 ... being fat reduces longevity: G. A. Gaesser, "Thinness and Weight Loss: Beneficial or Detrimental to Longevity?" *Medicine & Science in Sports & Exercise* 31 (8), 1118–28, 1999.

6. Buying Food and Eating Out

193 My sourcebook on food additives: Nancy and Edwardo Balingasa, *The Food Jungle: Your Self-Help Guide to Safe and Healthy Eating* (The Woodlands, Texas: Printed Matters, 1999), pp. 51–52.

198 ... organically grown fruits and vegetables: Bob L. Smith, "Organic Foods versus Supermarket Foods: Element Levels," *Journal of Applied Nutrition* 45 (1), 35–37, 1993.

199 ... verse from Lao Tzu: *The Way of Life According to Lao Tzu,* translated by Witter Bynner (New York: Perigee Books, 1972), p. 63.

Appendix D

278 Paramahansa Yogananda: Paramahansa Yogananda, *Autobiography of a Yogi* (Los Angeles: Self-Realization Fellowship, 1946), pp. 460–71.

ACKNOWLEDGMENTS

Once again I am grateful for the help of The Team: Sonny Mehta, Jonathan Segal, and Paul Bogaards at Alfred A. Knopf, and Richard Pine at Arthur Pine Associates. They provided inspiration and guidance in the creation of this book, from idea to reality. I also acknowledge the efforts of Richard Baxter and Michele Hardin in organizing my office and schedule so that I had time to write.

My medical partner, Dr. Brian Becker, helped me research the material for this book and track down references. He also made many editorial suggestions that I have incorporated. Jessica Pitluk also worked hard to gather references, and both she and Brian Becker got a great deal of assistance from Kathy Grant at the University of Arizona College of Pharmacy. Other research and editorial assistance came from Kathleen Johnson, Gary Nabhan, Si Reichlin, Dan Shapiro, and Cyndi Thomson.

A number of people contributed recipes. Marilyn Abraham of Santa Fe, New Mexico, developed a great many of them. Others came from Barbara Ruth Cohen (Asparagus Soup, Yellow Pepper and Carrot Soup, Zucchini Watercress Soup), Debra Dubois (Fruit "Pizza"), Elly Lewis (Pickled Carrots), Rita Rosenberg (Summer Melon Soup), and Betty Anne Sarver (Mushroom Barley Soup). All recipes were tested by Judith Berger and Suzan Gross of Culinary Concepts in Tucson, Arizona, and Suzan Gross did the nutritional analyses that follow the recipes.

I thank Nina Simonds, Dan Fields, and the staff of my *Self-Healing* newsletter for help in compiling the information in Appendix E. I also thank the Fellows and staff of the Program in Integrative Medicine for their support and encouragement, and Betty Anne and Diana for making me happy.

Andrew Weil
Tucson, Arizona
November 1999

INDEX

PROGRAM IN INTEGRATIVE MEDICINE

Dr. Andrew Weil directs the Program in Integrative Medicine at the University of Arizona College of Medicine. The mission of the Program is to redesign medical education to incorporate the philosophy of Integrative Medicine. The vision is this: to create a new kind of medicine, one that is based on a model of health rather than disease, one that trains practitioners to take the time to listen, to value nutritional and other lifestyle influences on health and illness, to offer treatments in addition to drugs and surgery, and to understand the innate potential of the human organism for self-repair and healing. Through training, research, and curriculum development, the Program educates physicians and other health care providers to realize the vision of Integrative Medicine both in clinical practice and in academic centers.

FOUNDATION FOR INTEGRATIVE MEDICINE

The Foundation for Integrative Medicine, established by Dr. Andrew Weil, is a non-profit, educational, and scientific organization dedicated to creating new paradigms of medicine for the twenty-first century. Gifts to the Foundation make possible the necessary research and training to ensure that the emerging field of Integrative Medicine will shape the future of health care.

For more information about PIM and FIM, please write to:

The Foundation for Integrative Medicine
1650 E. Fort Lowell Road
Suite 250
Tucson, Arizona 85719